BACK UP

Why back pain treatments aren't working and the new science offering hope

LIAM MANNIX

NEWSOUTH

A NewSouth book

Published by
NewSouth Publishing
University of New South Wales Press Ltd
University of New South Wales
Sydney NSW 2052
AUSTRALIA
https://unsw.press/

© Liam Mannix 2023
First published 2023

10 9 8 7 6 5 4 3 2 1

A catalogue record for this book is available from the National Library of Australia

ISBN   9781742238081 (paperback)
        9781742238791 (ebook)
        9781742239736 (ePDF)

Internal design Josephine Pajor-Markus
Cover design Akiko Chan
Cover image iStock, Ilbusca

BACK UP

Liam Mannix is a multi-award-winning national science reporter for *The Age* and the *Sydney Morning Herald*, as well as Nine's other stable of mastheads. He won the 2022 Press Club Quill Award for Excellence in Science, Medical and Health Reporting, the 2020 Walkley Award for Short Feature Writing, the 2019 Eureka Prize for Science Journalism, the 2019 Barry Williams Award for Skeptical Journalism and has twice won the Walkley Young Journalist of the Year (Innovation) award. He lives in Melbourne.

Forget everything you think you know about back pain. This book will do your head in, which is exactly what needs to happen. That's where the answers lie.

Dr Norman Swan, medical journalist and host of ABC Radio's *Health Report*

Back pain is the leading cause of disability in Australia and this book argues that this need not be the case. When the biggest predictor of chronic back pain is job satisfaction, something is wrong with our anatomic, mechanistic understanding of this common condition. *Back Up* sets the record straight by confronting our current understanding of pain, and chronic pain in particular.

Ian Harris, Professor of Orthopaedic Surgery and co-author of *Surgery, the Ultimate Placebo: A surgeon cuts through the evidence*

Back Up is an important book for anyone with chronic pain to read. It illustrates how too much medicine is significantly harming patients, rather than helping them. It should be a wake-up call for health professionals and patients.

Sophie Scott, Adjunct Associate Professor in Science Communication and former ABC national medical reporter

This bold and engaging investigative book by Liam Mannix will have you questioning what you thought you knew about the back, and how we experience and treat pain.

Aisha Dow, health editor with *The Age*

Contents

Foreword

Professor Chris Maher
The University of Sydney

Before considering Liam Mannix's book, *Back Up*, it is probably helpful to offer an introduction to back pain to set the scene.

Low back pain is the number-one cause of disability worldwide, affecting an estimated 540 million people at any point in time. In Australia, low back pain costs the Australian health system $4.8 billion annually and is the most common health reason forcing middle-aged Australians to retire early. This reduces Australia's GDP by more than $10.5 billion annually and can cause long-term financial hardship for individuals. For example, women forced to retire early due to low back pain reach the age of 65 with 10 per cent less wealth than their peers who remained in the workforce.

While we now have a good understanding for how low back pain should be managed, many people with this condition continue to receive poor healthcare – either missing out on recommended treatments or receiving treatments that are discouraged. And this confusing state is super expensive. The most costly surgical procedure in the US, at almost $US13 billion per year, is an unproven surgery for back pain. And yes, it is the very same surgery (well, one of them) that a certain famous golfer underwent.

Against this background it is understandable that someone would want to write a book on back pain for the everyday reader. In fact, many authors have, but the books are often terrible. The typical problem is that they are long on anecdotes and opinions, and short on science. *Back Up* is different and this would come as no surprise if you had met the author.

I first met Liam before he received his Eureka Prize for Science Journalism and his Walkley Award. But even without those awards, I quickly realised Liam was a different type of journalist. He asked a lot of questions, and when I sent him research papers to read he came back with even more questions. I am used to lots of questions as my main job is to supervise research students, but I had never had so many questions from a journalist. It was surprising and actually quite enjoyable.

And it was not just me that thought highly of Liam. Lots of my research colleagues had similarly positive encounters with him. So, when I learnt that he was writing this book I had pretty high expectations, and I was not disappointed when I received the first draft. Liam had spoken to the world's leading back pain researchers and intertwined those perspectives with his father's back pain story and his own back pain experience.

Liam is a great storyteller and a great science journalist, so *Back Up* is a fantastic read. There is stuff here that will surprise you and shock you, stuff that will make you angry and stuff that will fill you with hope. The story of back pain is not simple and the value of *Back Up* is that Liam has made that story accessible to the general reader. There is no other book like it if you want to understand the complexities around back pain.

A short detour to consider another condition that you would have heard of might help you appreciate why back pain is complex.

In medicine, the term 'syndrome' is used to describe a group of characteristic symptoms that co-occur; and when we also understand the cause and treatments we use the word 'disease' to describe the health condition.

When AIDS (Acquired Immunodeficiency Syndrome) was first described in 1981, its cause was a complete mystery. But within a few years it was discovered that the syndrome was due to a viral infection. In contrast, we have known about back pain for thousands of years – even Hippocrates wrote about it. However, even with 2500 years of recognition, we are still mainly stuck at the syndrome stage for back pain that we were with AIDS in 1981.

Sadly, for 95 per cent of patients with back pain, we don't know why they experience it. This is enormously frustrating for the patient, and also the clinician. The treatments we have for back pain can only target the symptoms, not the cause, and so the best treatments we have are only modestly effective. And yet in many cases, for a whole range of complex reasons, patients are missing out on these known treatments. Instead, in some settings, what is actually more common is ineffective and harmful care.

So what has gone wrong? Well, it's complicated, and the value of Liam Mannix's book is how he explains it. Liam walks us through the myths and misunderstandings about low back pain, exposes how vested interests have conspired to create an epidemic of poor care, and illustrates how much suffering this epidemic of poor care has inflicted on individuals and society.

But there is hope and *Back Up* offers this beautifully – revealing a way forward out of this mess. It provides people with back pain the knowledge they need to navigate a complex health system so that they are more likely to receive the right care and recover. Liam covers the new science of pain – and how we think about and conceptualise our pain – opening the way for new ways of viewing and managing back pain. He explains that our backs are strong and capable and that they thrive on movement. He uses the science, and the examples of his father's and his own back pain, to illustrate that recovery from back pain is within our own control.

Introduction
The curse of a bad back

My dad has had a bad back for as long as I can remember.

It has cast a long shadow over his life and the life of my family. It strained our family and put him through years of pain during what should have been the best years of his life. He can't remember chunks because of the heavy-duty painkillers he was eating like candy. At his darkest points, he thought he might not walk again. He spent a week in a pain clinic. We had paramedics round to the house. He collapsed in a restaurant. He contemplated suicide. We moved states because of that damn back.

After years of agony, Dad had disc surgery. Afterwards, his surgeon paid him a bedside visit to tell him that, yes, as suspected, one of his discs had been protruding into the sciatic nerve that runs down the leg. The nerve was red and inflamed, the surgeon said. With the disc's edge lopped off, the fissure sealed with surgical cement, the pressure on the nerve would ease and the pain would go away within a few months.

And, slowly, the pain went away, and it stayed away. After years of pain, of whole weekends ruined because of a crook back, suddenly I had a Dad who could walk again – who could run again, who could play basketball again. It was a bit of a miracle, really, or like the lifting of a curse in a fairytale. I was pretty sure the grass was gleaming greener as we strolled down to the basketball court for the first time in a long time, me, Dad, my sister.

The surgery worked. But here's the thing: it shouldn't have. A wide range of back pain experts told me they would never recommend surgery in Dad's case. One described it as 'criminal'.

I've suffered from back pain all my life, although it's never been as bad as Dad's. After seeing what Dad went through, I was committed to finding a way to make sure it never would be. But as I dug into the science of back pain, interviewing patients and doctors and scientific experts, a very strange story started to emerge. Back pain, I discovered, is an epidemic of extraordinary scale. About four million Australians will have it every year; about 175 000 will be hospitalised.[1] And the problem seems to be getting worse, not better – despite, or possibly because of, the enormous sums of money we spend on it.

And the way we treat it seems to be seriously messed up. Most treatments simply don't work, or aren't supported by the science. Many of them are extortionately expensive and pose real risks, yet because of vested interests we keep giving them to people.

But more than this classic tale of medical malpractice, what intrigued me about back pain was a strange theory that had started to emerge in the last 20 years. One that suggested both doctors and society at large had gotten the way we think about back pain, and pain in general, all wrong. This radical theory suggests that much pain is driven in part not by anything wrong with our backs but something wrong with our culture and our ideas and how we *think* about pain. An idea as a virus. A social disease.

This theory suggested that surgery did not cure Dad's back. It cured his thinking.

Professor James McAuley leans forward and starts talking fast, like he knows you won't believe him unless he gets all the words out quickly. Which, to be fair, I don't. His attire today isn't helping: spiked hair, bushy moustache, wire-frame glasses, a black hoodie with too-long sleeves he keeps picking at, all which suggest a cross between mad scientist and sullen teenager.

'What do we think about backs in our Western culture?' he asks me. I kind of get the sense he's not really interested in my answer, so I stay mute. 'We think they often get fragile as you get a bit older. And they're not very strong, really. We think you should sit up straight most of the time. And it's something that really should be protected.'

We think you should lift with a straight back, he says. We think posture is important. We think ergonomics is a thing. We think we should strengthen our core, lift with our abs. We think the spine, the discs, are fragile. We think you can slip a disc. We think backs can be hurt so bad, you'd never be the same.

None of that – *none of that* – is true, says McAuley.

I sit in McAuley's office, stunned. I've had back pain for years, caused by a slipped disc. And now here's James McAuley, one of the world's leading experts on back pain, *telling me you can't slip a disc?*

McAuley is kind enough to look almost apologetic. 'You can't,' he tells me. 'It's … it's just not true. None of the evidence suggests it's true.'

It is the western world's cultural beliefs, McAuley says, that have got us where we are: a world in which back pain is now the leading cause of disability in most countries,[2] where people seem to be getting sicker despite no detectable cause of illness, where billions are spent on cures that make us sicker. 'In fact,' he says, 'the more you worry about that stuff, the more likely you are to get back pain.'

McAuley is angry and energised. He is not alone, I've come to learn. Many, many of the leading back pain scientists around the world feel like this. They believe back pain is one of the greatest problems in world health today. And it is one almost entirely of our own creation.

'If we stopped all back pain treatment, all of it,' another leading scientist would later tell me, 'we could halve the amount of back pain in the world. *Halve*. And we could do it tomorrow.'

What you'll find in this book is the result of several years of interviewing leading experts on back and chronic pain across Australia.

Chronic back pain is a subset of the even wider problem of chronic pain, which overall is the largest cause of disease and disability worldwide. One in five Australians has chronic pain. This ranges from chronic headaches to arthritis and endometriosis. There are many differences between them, and many things in common – like the common experience of one's pain not being believed. And they present a growing threat, with GP presentations for chronic pain up 67 per cent in the last decade in Australia.

But among these conditions, it is low back pain that is consistently the leading cause of years lived with disability.

As you've seen, this book begins with a personal story, mine and my dad's. Then it looks at the back itself, whether it's a weak spot, whether we're simply built wrong, why so many people seem to have back pain. Then we'll look at some of the pieces of common knowledge about our backs that turn out to be wildly off base. We'll investigate several expensive back pain treatments, look at the science, meet the people who've gone under the knife and hear their stories. This is the old science of back pain.

The second half of the book focuses on the new science. How neuroscience has revolutionised the way scientists think about pain and what that can tell us about sore backs. How the crucial connection between brain and back can break down, and how to rebuild it.

Finally, we'll tour rehab approaches with the best evidence behind them, to see how we can all build stronger, pain-free backs.

1   The extent of the problem

How many people like my dad are out there? How big is the back pain problem?

Stunningly enormous.

It is 'one of the biggest problems for public health systems in the western world,' venerable medical journal the *Lancet* notes.[1] 'And now it seems to be extending worldwide.' As many as 84 per cent of us will suffer from back pain at some time in our lives. In Australia, one in six people have back pain every year – almost 4 million people. It will put about 180000 Australians in hospital. Back problems are the leading health burden for Australians aged 45 to 74, and our second biggest burden overall behind heart problems. Think about that for a moment: of all the ills that ail Australians, like mental health or diabetes, back pain takes the most healthy life away from us. It is the fifth-leading reason why adults end up in emergency departments in Australia.

And of everyone who gets back pain, between 10 and 15 per cent will develop chronic back pain.[2] These are crazy numbers. In Australia, we spend about $1.7 billion in direct public and private hospital costs on back problems; one paper put the costs associated with lower back pain in the US at $100 to $200 billion a year.[3] European Union researchers estimated it cost the Union 1.5 per cent of GDP a year in lost productivity. In Australia, back problems cost our health system at least $4.7 billion a year. That's not counting the huge burden of all these working-age people taken out of society and stuck on disability pensions, nor the enormous emotional toll of all that pain.

And it's getting worse. Globally, the number of people with back pain continues to increase.[4] The number of Australians heading to hospital with back pain has increased in the last decade, while the people sitting in emergency with 'non-acute' back pain – garden variety back pain – has tripled in number in that time. The percentage of Australians who have self-reported long-term chronic back and disc issues rose from 6.4 per cent to 15.1 per cent between 1995 and 2004–2005.[5]

It has now reached such epidemic proportions, we need to start fighting it with the same alarm with which we fight cancer, asthma and heart disease, says Curtin University back pain expert Professor Andrew Briggs. And here's the truly pernicious bit. 'The amount we spend, and the amount of services we offer, that's going up, but at the same time, disability is increasing,' he tells me. 'We're spending more, doing more stuff, but it's not helping.'

Scientists have never known more about back pain. We spend billions each year trying to treat it, largely for naught. Something is badly, badly wrong.

One expensive 'fix' – spinal cord stimulators

Izzy Sulejmani has two spinal cord stimulators, each worth about $25 000, wired into his back.

Each small box has five electric wires that worm through Sulejmani's tissues and terminate at his nerves. At the command of a computer program, electricity flows silently from the box, down the leads, and out into Sulejmani's back, neck and shoulders. The theory – and no one knows for sure, because no one is truly sure how they work – is the electricity interferes with the nerves in Sulejmani's body that are causing him pain.

They weren't implanted at the same time. The man who put them there told Sulejmani the first might help with his back, neck and shoulder pain. It did not. So the man put a second one in. Each device costs around $35 000 – plus another $8000 in doctor and hospital fees, plus *another* $18 000 for the trial every patient must undertake.

The second device worked better, but the first box still sat under the skin and did nothing at all.

When we spoke in mid-2019 Sulejmani had a question for me: do I think he should get another one?

Because that's what his pain specialist was now offering him, and the pain was so bad but the other stimulators only seem to make things worse, and he didn't know what to do. I sucked in a breath, and told him I didn't know what he should do either.

'The surgeon that put them in, I kept telling him I needed them fixed. But for some reason he kept blaming me, and saying it was my fault,' Sulejmani told me. 'I thought I was the only one. The way my pain specialist was talking to me, it was like I was the only one with these problems. The more I was trying to get it fixed, the worse I was being treated.'

The stimulators shocked him. They regularly seemed

to misfire, sending electrical shocks coursing through his body. The batteries needed regular recharging, which you do by sticking a magnetic charger to the skin surface over the device. The charger heated up, burning Sulejmani's skin. He called the salesman from the huge medical device company that makes and sells the charger, the one who was in the operating theatre when Sulejmani's doctor put it in, and asked him what to do. Try an icepack, he was told. 'I cannot control the stimulation. Say I've got it on two, and I move, it jumps up to a ten. It's not a very good feeling, not a very good feeling at all,' he said.

Sulejmani's back pain story started with a tingling in his arm. Some of the nerves for the arm feed down from the brain, along the spinal cord, and out along the limb. Izzy's doctors thought one of his spinal discs – C5–C6, the disc between the two vertebrae that you can feel at the base of your neck – was bulging and trapping a nerve. They operated on the disc. 'It did not work,' says Sulejmani. The surgeon then opted to go back in, removing the disc and replacing it with a system of screws and rods to hold the spine in place. That worked a bit better. Then Sulejmani got caught in a car accident. The impact left him with lasting pain in his neck, shoulder and back.

'I did not want to have any operations. I tried everything,' Sulejmani told me. 'Yoga, Pilates. The only thing I did not try was hypnosis. But the pain ended up getting that bad that I went and had the spinal fusion. Which I shouldn't have had done.'

Sulejmani ended up with fusions at two separate points in his spine. Neither worked. They gave him drugs for the pain – morphine. He became addicted. Sulejmani sent me a thick sheaf of correspondence between him, his surgeon and the health department. Complaints and rejections. The stimulators were working just as they should be, the department told him at one point. 'Nothing has improved,' Sulejmani wrote on one of the forms in blue ballpoint pen. 'THEY DON'T WORK'.

In January 2015, a 49-year-old man sat down to write a letter to his government. It was all he could think to do. He had a Medtronic RestoreSensor Model 37714 implanted in his back, with wires fed into his spinal cord, to treat the back pain he'd had since having his spine fused a decade prior. Price: $20 000. At first, the system seemed to be working, he wrote. Then it broke. The machine, which is built to pulse low-frequency electricity into the spine, turned itself up and just started shocking him repeatedly, 'painfully and uncontrollably'.

'If I was not home at this time to reach the remote control this would have been a torturous pain that I could not have stopped until the device was turned off,' he wrote. Three painful surgeries to correct the problem, and it still wasn't fixed. The wires seemed to have detached and were moving freely around his spine, causing excruciating pain.

Eventually, the doctor – not a surgeon, the author noted – who put the device in agreed to take it out. At the clinic for his operation, the man watched the Medtronic representative head into the doctor's surgery first, ignoring him. 'I realise,' the man wrote, 'that this company was just using me. The fact that the Medtronic people showed no concern and made me feel like a worthless guinea pig leaves me with a feeling of hopelessness and helplessness as to my future and quality of life.'

He was on disability and had, he wrote, no idea how he was going to pay for the cost of the reoperation. Exhausted, the only thing he could do was pen a letter to an anonymous government inbox. 'No one else should ever have to go through the pain and suffering that I have,' he wrote. And then, tacked on to the bottom of the note:

New update

X ray on 1/6/2015 shows doctor FORGOT to remove 6 inch lead that is still inside me now torturously starting to protrude from my skin.

Please help ASAP

I stared at this message when I found it buried within an obscure government database that collects medical complaints. 'Reviewed', the database noted at the end of the complaint. 'No further action needed.'

There were more like it.

'Since I have had it in, I have had six revisions,' wrote another patient who was also given a Medtronic RestoreSensor. 'Surely this can't be right … All these procedures, the trauma and the pain. What am I to do? I don't know who to talk to or get advice. Do I need legal advice?' The unnamed patient noted he was suffering from incontinence. The database noted that 'no further action [was] required'.

Between 2012 and 2019 the Therapeutic Goods Administration, Australia's medical regulator, received 520 reports of serious injuries linked to spinal cord stimulators. To give you a sense of how high that number is, compare it to pelvic mesh, which turned into a medical device regulation scandal. The TGA received about 100 reports of serious injuries related to pelvic mesh before it launched an inquiry.

'Five hundred and twenty-five is a heck of a lot,' Danny Vadasz, former chief executive of the Health Issues Centre and the campaigner who has spearheaded the campaign that turned mesh into a scandal, told me. 'That's enough for a class action.' And stimulators are implanted a lot less often than mesh.

Nearly all reports on the TGA database I was looking at come from the device manufacturers themselves – who have a strong and obvious incentive not to report problems. A 2019 analysis by the TGA's own staff suggest just 0.5 per cent of all problems may end up being reported – meaning 520 is a vast under-exaggeration.[6] In America, spinal cord stimulators have the third-highest medical device injury reports made to the US Food and Drug Administration. Stimulators were once an option of last resort for people with chronic pain. They are increasingly being sold as a high-tech, low-risk first resort for people with all sorts of pain, including back pain.

Bill (who asked I not use his real name) was not in extreme pain when he had one installed. He had nagging pain – four out of ten, perhaps. He hadn't tried anything. His pain specialist installed a spinal cord stimulator anyway. Initially the stimulator did little to help his pain, so it was turned up. 'It felt like someone was poking me with a hot poker,' says Bill. He called his device representative. 'They say, if it's hurting, turn it up.' He refused, and turned it off. Later, his installer told him a lead had moved. 'I found absolutely no pain relief. None. If anything, it aggravated the area. This is what I would say to people: be careful with your levels,' he says.

Lauren Iacobucci did receive good relief from her stimulator at first. But then, after a fall, she felt the electrodes come out of her spine. 'I had surgery to fix the leads, and then they became displaced again. A month after that surgery, I had another surgery to fix them again. And then the wound just wouldn't heal. It just kept opening up and the leads would just pop through my skin.'

Mrs Iacobucci had six surgeries in total before she gave up and demanded the device be removed. 'It was horrendous. I can't describe it. It's only recently I've started processing what I went through.'

Adam Young, 54, keeps his spinal cord stimulator in his kitchen cupboard. He got it to fix his injured back. It did nothing for the pain. 'He just kept giving me the bullshit story: it will get better, it will get better. Now I got a $40 000 stimulator sitting in my cupboard that I can use as a party trick. That's it. It's just a big waste of time, and an absolute money grab.'

The biggest issue with the devices appears to be their propensity to move. Either the stimulator itself – usually attached near the hip – wanders from its surgical pocket, or the leads detach and move through the back. In various studies this ranges from 0.3 per cent all the way up to 14 per cent.[7] Reoperation rates run up to 31 per cent.

'Thirty per cent, for a reasonable human being, seems

really high,' says Dr Chris Hayes, director of the Hunter Integrated Pain Service and a former dean of the Faculty of Pain Medicine at the Australian and New Zealand College of Anaesthetists.

Early in his career, Dr Hayes regularly implanted spinal cord stimulators. He no longer performs the procedure. 'We decided the outcomes were not good. We were getting quite a few take-backs to theatre. Patient harm. With stimulators, it's not that uncommon for the lead to move – then you have to take the patient back to theatre and put the lead back to where it's meant to be. And these devices can get infected. We found a reasonably high complication rate, even trying to be very careful.'

Dr Hayes published a study of six patients who had been given stimulators for back pain. 'And they were all hugely better off without the stimulators. Maybe there's a place for stimulators, in very select patients. But we're saying, given the current evidence, we're not offering that treatment at this point in time.'

I find the case studies of stimulator injury, recorded in cold bureaucratic language in the government regulators' database, chilling:

- Multiple patients who experienced weakness in the legs and temporarily lost the ability to walk.
- One patient's knees gave way and they hit their head on the ground. They were placed in an induced coma in hospital.
- Three patients lost the use of their legs until the stimulator was removed. Another lost feeling in their

pelvis. Another had 'arm weakness' – an MRI showed spinal damage.

- Multiple patients suffered from incontinence for long periods of time.
- Multiple patients suffered tears and punctures to the sheath covering their spinal cord. Another suffered cerebrospinal fluid leakage. Another suffered a spinal cord tear which caused incontinence.
- One patient suffered a haemorrhage leading to seizures, while two others suffered uncontrollable muscle spasms.
- Two patients developed infection at the surgery site, which caused multiple organ failure in one and sepsis in the other, killing them. Another suffered a stroke due to spending a long time in the operating theatre, and died.

Then there were more common side effects: over-stimulation, constantly being shocked, the stimulation not working, device malfunction, headaches, infection, pain at the surgical site, or the leads detaching from the spine and moving around in the body or protruding through the skin. Most cases on the database required a second surgery to correct. Many require several.

'I think there are a lot of stimulators being put in inappropriately,' says Dr Michael Johnson, president of the Spine Society of Australia between 2018 and 2020.

'In the last year, I've operated on three people ... and taken out a stimulator and thrown it in the bin. That's a pretty substantial investment to just throw in the bin. And none of these people had received an opinion from a spinal surgeon.'

Dr Nick Christelis, an installer and spokesman for the Neuromodulation Society of Australia and New Zealand, told me the devices came with only 'minor risks'. Studies showing higher rates of complications were based on older devices, and anaesthetists were better at installing them now, he said. 'The complication rate is about one in 10 over the lifespan of the device. Which could be anything from a little bit of discomfort to where the battery lies, to full blown infection requiring removal.'

A spokeswoman for the TGA told me that the reports of incidents associated with use of medical devices does not necessarily mean that the device was at fault and the cause of the incident.

'Spinal cord stimulators, used quite widely both in Australia and worldwide, are high-risk devices and are known to have complications associated with their use,' the spokeswoman said.

'The current information indicates that the safety and performance of these devices are acceptable. The TGA continues to monitor adverse event reports associated with these types of devices.'

I handed the database to Professor Chris Maher. Based at the University of Sydney, Maher is founding director of the government-funded Institute for Musculoskeletal Health; he and I have worked together on several back pain investigations. He was intrigued, and asked one of his talented PhD students, Caitlin Jones, to take a look.

Of the 520 events in the database, Jones and her team classified 93 as serious or life-threatening. More than half were caused by the stimulator itself malfunctioning. Some 79 per cent of events required surgery to correct. Jones concluded that spinal cord stimulators had more than double the risk of adverse events compared to pacemakers, even though pacemaker operations affect the heart, while spinal cord stimulators are meant to be low-impact. For every 100 stimulators inserted, 31 are later removed, according to Medicare data – which compares to just two out of every 100 pacemakers.

Data I obtained from private insurers is even more damning: 40.8 per cent of Australians who receive a stimulator will have another hospital operation – likely to the stimulator – within three years. For a hip or knee replacement that figure is about 1.5 per cent. One health fund patient got two stimulators, and then needed two reoperations within the next two years, at a total cost of $236385; another had six stimulator replacements in four years at an eyewatering $400000-plus.

How do such troubled devices get approved? Sometimes through a loophole.

The US Food and Drug Administration is viewed as one of the world's gold standard medical device regulators. Its judgements carry enormous weight for other, smaller regulators like our own TGA. And for years the FDA had been allowing new spinal cord stimulators to be approved through a loophole, an investigation by the Associated Press revealed in 2018.[8]

Initial approval for a device may be rigorous. But once that's achieved, device companies can use so-called 'supplementary requests' to alter their products – avoiding major scrutiny, even when the changes are major. There were just six new spinal cord stimulators approved by the FDA since 1984, the AP found, and 835 supplemental changes. Devices are rarely pulled from the market, even when serious problems emerged.

Australia's own TGA – whose entire budget comes from pharmaceutical and device companies – says it does not accept spinal cord stimulators approved through the FDA's loophole. However, it does not do its own testing of medical devices before approval, leaving that up to the manufacturer. Nor does it keep a register of devices implanted in Australia.

This leaves it in a strange situation. In 2012 a batch of Eon Mini spinal cord stimulators was recalled by the FDA due to what it described as 'sudden, brief surge[s] in stimulation'. Rather than following suit, the TGA issued a 'hazard notice', noting battery issues. The agency said this was because – in what must be regarded as medical regulator irony – they couldn't be recalled because they had all been inserted inside patients.

The faulty stimulator lots that were shocking patients in America hadn't been supplied in Australia, the regulator told me. 'They wouldn't know that,' says Danny Vadasz. 'Because they don't have a register.'

Between 2012 and 2019 I found 66 reports of side effects in the TGA's database linked to the Eon Mini, 13 of them involving overshocking. One patient reported electrical shocks through his whole body, making it hard to breathe. Another reporting the shocking making it difficult to stand – he fell over and was injured.

In 2014, the TGA issued a recall notice – for the Eon

Mini's charger, after several patients were burned by it overheating. The whole device's medical registration was cancelled by the device's sponsor in 2016, the TGA said.

It's important to note that the huge companies that sell the stimulators have close financial ties to the doctors installing the devices, the scientists studying them, and the charities meant to represent patients.

An army of sales staff is employed to spruik these expensive devices, some of whom can earn up to US$600 000 a year.[9] The big financial incentives involved have led some to bend the rules: in 2015 Medtronic paid the US government US$2.8 million to settle claims that it encouraged doctors to submit false healthcare claims and pushed pain doctors to install spinal cord stimulators in chronic pain cases where they weren't indicated. Medtronic allegedly told physicians they could 'make upward of $10 000 profit on each patient, while adding only minutes to the procedure'.

And the sales staff appear to have a very close relationship with patients. Every single patient I spoke to said a representative from a device company was in the room during their surgery. Often they, not the doctors, advise patients on how to adjust the stimulators. Most had follow-up treatment provided by the company representative, often without a doctor present. If problems arose, some were told to call their device representative first, rather than their doctor. A Boston Scientific job ad for a Queensland manager notes the successful applicant will do device programming and patient follow-up, as well as achieving sales targets.

One patient told me he had a stimulator trial – where the leads are implanted but the stimulator is not – and was left in agony after a lead moved. The sales representative kept pushing him to keep trying with the stimulator, even as his own doctor agreed it wasn't working. 'The representative was a complete bastard,' he told me. 'Once he knew [there was] no money to be made from me, man, he showed his true colours. The amount of persuasive rhetoric he tried … Totally heartless people.'

The Australian Pain Management Association bills itself as a charity set up to advocate for and support Australians living with pain. But it also helps sell spinal cord stimulators, which it describes as 'less invasive than surgery'. 'Because of this, the complications are reduced.'

In late 2018, APMA launched a national roadshow to educate Australians living with chronic pain called 'Taking back control of my chronic pain'. 'The Australian Pain Management Association (APMA) invites you to attend a FREE seminar specifically for Australians living with chronic pain, their families, and carers,' a website linked to the campaign read.

The clue everything was not quite as it seemed was all the way down the bottom of the website. Brought to you by … Boston Scientific. The website's privacy policy listed a privacy policy for Boston Scientific websites, while the terms of use simply read 'Welcome to www.bostonscientific.com'. The company was not mentioned on the invite to the event, distributed under APMA's letterhead. Who really was running this roadshow? The star speaker was Justin Minyard, a retired US Army master sergeant who according to his LinkedIn account was working as a neuromodulation consultant for Boston Scientific at the time of the roadshow.

The charity received $50 625 in grants in 2018, making up nearly all its small budget. It raised just $195 in donations.

A spokeswoman for APMA told me the organisation 'does not endorse any particular medical treatment for chronic pain', and had never received any sponsorship from Boston Scientific.

'Our records indicate that APMA was a speaker at the event and was remunerated for speaking fees of $1500,' she said.

This seemed to raise further questions. 'I'm confused. I thought it was your event? Was it actually Boston Scientific's event, and you were paid as a speaker?' I wrote back. The spokeswoman did not reply – and Boston Scientific declined to comment when contacted for this book.

Medtronic's tentacles reach deep. The Neuromodulation Society of Australia and New Zealand, the peak body for spinal cord stimulation, boldly proclaim that stimulators are 'a minimally-invasive and reversible therapy that may prove an effective, additional or alternative option for those who have tried and failed conservative pain management options'. That claim is based in part on a widely cited and influential 2011 Australian review that recommends who should receive a stimulator.[10] The review was sponsored by Medtronic.

As a sign of how influential that company-sponsored review is, the Australian and New Zealand College of Anaesthetists (ANZCA) – Australia's peak body for pain medicine – referenced the review in professional information it supplied to its pain medicine fellows. Medtronic paid $63 900 to the college between 2017 and 2019 to exhibit at the college's annual scientific meeting, and another $12 870 to support the college's 'refresher course day'. The college has also received payments from Abbott, Boston Scientific and Nevro, who all make and sell stimulators.

'ANZCA is meticulous in its approach to managing real or potential conflicts of interest. Content and speakers are approved/vetted by the scientific convenor of meetings and workshops and all presenters are required to declare any potential conflicts of interest,' a college spokeswoman told me.

Despite almost 60 years of practice implanting stimulators, the community of medicos who install them are still not absolutely sure how they work. It was first thought the electrical pulses block pain signals from being sent to the brain, but that theory did not hold up. Proponents now believe they might work by doing that, or by stimulating a big influx of painkilling chemicals, or by changing the nervous system itself. 'It does a lot of different things. We know there are many different ways it works. We just don't know the main way, the number one way,' Dr Christelis from the Neuromodulation Society tells me. Nevertheless, 'Nowadays, with the new technology, we can expect up to 80 per cent pain control or more,' he says.

When I first published an investigation of stimulators in *The Age* in early 2022, it was difficult to prove that 'up to 80 per cent' claim true or false. The evidence for spinal cord stimulators was patchy and confusing. Some trials seemed to show terrific results ... but they were industry funded. Others tested different patterns of stimulation against each other. Some registered huge numbers of patient harms, others relatively few. Other studies secretly turned off the stimulators – and showed that, in fact, the patients felt no more pain, suggesting a large placebo effect. 'How well they work – or whether they work at all – remains deeply controversial,' I wrote.

A year later, as I write this, that evidence base has changed.

In October, *JAMA* published a study of 50 patients in Norway left with chronic pain after spinal surgery.[11] Each patient had a stimulator implanted, then spent six months with it turned on, and – without the patient knowing – another six months with it essentially turned off. It made no difference. The researchers found there were no significant differences in scores for pain, disability or quality of life, whether the stimulator was on or off.

'This study ... doesn't remotely represent what we do for our patients and doesn't reflect the clinical outcome that we see in our patients,' Neuromodulation Society of Australia and New Zealand president Dr James Yu told me.

But to the Institute for Musculoskeletal Health's Dr Adrian Traeger, who is working on a Cochrane review of the evidence for spinal cord stimulators to treat back pain, 'This is a strong signal this treatment may not work.'

A quick note on Cochrane, because they are important in this book. An independent, not-for-profit foundation, Cochrane pulls together the world's best experts to thoroughly review scientific evidence. Was the study conducted correctly? Was the trial designed such that the scientists' own biases and beliefs interfered with the results? Was it funded by someone who stood to gain from a particular outcome? They tell you what the evidence is, and how believable that evidence is. Scientists commonly consider a Cochrane review to be the gold standard for scientific evidence. I'll refer to their work frequently in this book.

Two Cochrane reviews, Traeger's upcoming paper and another by a UK-led team published in 2021, also found low-quality evidence to suggest spinal cord stimulators work no better than a placebo.[12]

Why are the Cochrane reviews so negative when some of the underlying studies are so positive? Because, Traeger told me, these studies are almost designed to mislead. They compare a stimulator to people getting 'usual medical care' – but that care is often deliberately bad, making the stimulator seem better by comparison. 'And they kick people who aren't improving with spinal cord stimulation out of the study but don't extend that courtesy to people who are not improving with usual medical care,' he says.

As I spent the last few years writing this book, and covering the blighted topic of back pain in the pages of *The Age* and the *Sydney Morning Herald*, I came across many stories like Izzy's. People who find a small pain in their back – a niggle they've ignored over the years, perhaps – slowly, slowly worsening until it becomes unbearable. They try everything they can themselves, but nothing helps. Then they turn, as we are taught to, to doctors and surgeons – where they often find themselves being prescribed treatments that are either experimental or shown not to work. Sometimes it makes things worse, or exposes patients to risks. Nearly always it costs a lot of money.

The story of how Izzy and many like him ended up with enormously expensive – yet, for many, ineffective – devices wired into their spines is a case study in everything that is sick in the way we treat back pain.

The trouble with backs

As I set out on my journey to understand what had gone so badly wrong, and why, I decided I needed to take a closer look at where all these problems began. I needed Paul McMenamin.

McMenamin, a professor and director of the Centre for Human Anatomy Education at Monash University, is an avuncular Scot who sounds just like Sean Connery. He is, I suspect, leaning into it. He loves James Bond – and in his new and fully kitted out anatomy lab he is a real-life Q.

Along one wall of McMenamin's lab runs a series of skeletons. The first is thick and quadrupedal, with a thick skull, huge jaw, hands firmly on the ground and a thick spine that terminates in a little stubby tail that reminds me of a pig's corkscrew.

He leads me along the wall and together we watch as the skeletons become progressively more upright. The pelvic bone tilts upwards at an awkward angle, the bones lengthen, the skull shrinks, and the face's Neanderthal features retreat. Eventually, I come face to face with a naked, grinning and very upright *Homo sapiens*.

McMenamin spins this last skeleton around to point at the bit that has remained central all the way through our family tree, from quadruped to biped: the spine.

The spine is made of 24 vertebrae – that's the bony bits you can feel with your hand – he says, indicating each with his fingers. If you could look inside the bones you'd see they were honeycomb, the genius bit of design that allows them to be both strong and light. Ounce for ounce, bone is stronger than steel.[13] To deal with the increased loads of standing upright, our vertebrae start out small in your neck and get progressively larger and stronger as they run down your spine.

In between each of those vertebrae sit intervertebral discs, which are hard on the outside and soft on the inside. The soft centre of the disc acts as a shock–distributor, spreading the load across the spine as you walk around.

On first glance, they look really thick. They spread right to the edges of the vertebrae. They look nothing like the hamburger patties, ready to slide out of the bun at the slightest touch, that I guess I was imagining. They don't look fragile. McMenamin nods. 'The outer ring of the disc is fibrous and really strong. You literally couldn't tear it apart with your bare hands.'

He beckons me closer. The cleverest bit of the design, he says, is right here. He jabs a finger at the point where each vertebra comes together at the back of the spine. It looks like a hinge. These hinges, called facet joints, combine with the discs to allow the spine to move. But each hinge is cut to a slightly different angle. In the lower back, the angles allow the vertebrae to bend right forward – that's how you touch your toes – and a little way back. Higher up, behind your rib cage, the angles are cut so you can twist side to side but can't really flex back and forward (go and test this for yourself!).

Each vertebra is joined to the next by ligaments – hard, elastic bands of tissue which give the spine its stiffness. Those ligaments are so strong it takes blunt force trauma to tear them – think a car accident. If you want to feel them, stand up and lean forward. When you can't bend forward any further, that's your spinal ligaments. You're hanging off them like a puppet.

Movement is created by the muscles of the spine and core. Long sheets of muscle on the back, next to the spine, allow you to bend forwards and back and side-to-side. Stabilising muscles sit in a ring around the entire body and help hold everything firm. The spine itself has little strength; it is the muscles that provide it. When all are sheared away, the spine itself can support just two kilograms.[14]

'The muscles act like struts,' says McMenamin. 'Imagine a building built of blocks, and the floor is connected like the discs – that building would be pretty unstable, but it has to be, because the building has to flop back and forward as you bend. It has to be unstable. The muscles are like big foam supports around the building to ensure it doesn't fall over.'

'So,' I say to McMenamin, 'which bit hurts when you have back pain?'

He screws up his face. He's an anatomy expert, not a back pain researcher. He wanders over to his model, waving a finger up and down the spine. There are plenty of things that can hurt, he says.

The vertebrae of the spine are hollow, with a neat hole that runs the length of the spine. Through that runs the spinal cord, the thick neural highway that carries all the information from your body to your brain and vice versa. If the discs or vertebrae shift out of alignment, they can pinch the nerves that emerge at each level between the vertebrae.

All the way down the spinal cord sprout cables of nerves which run off and into the limbs, allowing you to send commands to your fingers and toes. These nerves run past the discs down the spine and exit through the foramina between the vertebrae, McMenamin says.

I bend down to look at the tiny hole that somehow appears between one hinge and the next: 'There's not a lot of room there.' 'No,' says McMenamin. 'There's not a lot of room. Add in the soft tissues, the ligaments, the blood vessels, the sheath around the nerve – there's no room ... It's very tight. It only takes a disc to bulge a mil [millimetre] or two and you'll get pain.'

The sacroiliac joints sit between the thick base of your spine and the hard bone of the pelvis, and allow you to tilt your torso backwards and forwards. Thick bunches of nerves run through here and down into the leg, and they can get caught up and damaged. And then there's all the soft tissue itself, which can be directly injured or fatigued from overwork.[15]

McMenamin's family tree is troubling. Our ancestors looked squat and strong as they spread the load between legs and arms. We, on the other hand, looked downright unwieldy. In early humans – and apes – the spine looks solid and straight. That pushes their centre of gravity forward, making an ape front-heavy. Babies have spines that look rather similar to apes', with two curves in them; they develop two more as they spend more time upright and less time rolling around on the floor. The mature human spine must support a bobbing head atop its stack, as well as provide structural integrity for the rest of the body.[16]

Is there something uniquely weak about all that anatomy? Are our backs simply badly designed? Some scientists think so.

'If you want one place cobbled together with duct tape and paper clips, it's the back,' anatomist and paleoanthropologist Bruce Latimer of Case Western Reserve University told the annual meeting of the American Association for the Advancement of Science in 2013.[17]

Latimer was speaking from the perspective of evolutionary history. Our ancestors, he reckoned, had much more robust spines than we do. Two Neanderthal spines found in caves in modern day Israel and Iraq don't show any significant signs of spinal degeneration – which surprised the scientists who studied them, who expected their brutally arduous lifestyles would have left a mark.[18] Our modern sedentary lifestyles mean our muscles and bones aren't exposed to as much stress as ancient hunter–gatherers, so they end up a lot weaker.[19] 'If you take care of it, your spine will get you through to about 40 or 50,' said Latimer. 'After that, you're on your own.'

However, there are plenty of people who don't buy this line of thinking.

People who complain the spine is poorly designed 'are often creationists', says Professor John Long, an expert in vertebrate palaeontology at Flinders University. 'Evolution usually does not make mistakes. If it's wrong, it doesn't work, and those species go extinct. The spine is perfectly adapted for what it was meant to do.'

And there's lots of evidence our spines are capable of feats of extreme strength. 'Look at weightlifters. The stuff your back does is incredible,' says Professor Chris Maher, who we met earlier, and who is one of the world's top back pain researchers. A badly designed spine didn't seem to stop Iceland's Hafþór Júlíus Björnsson deadlifting 501 kilograms in 2020 to take the Guinness World Record. Deadlifters bend at the waist, flatten their back, and reach down to pick up huge loads. As they stand, a lot of stress goes through the vertebrae. They don't break. An Olympic weightlifter can put more than 6700 Newtons of force through their L5–S1 joint during a Romanian deadlift,[20] yet weightlifters actually suffer fewer injuries than people playing contact sports, a 2016 review found.[21]

If back pain was caused by a fundamental weakness in our backs, we'd know, because the whole experience of back pain would be entirely different, argues Maher. Why do most people tend to feel better a few weeks after injuring their back? And why is it only a smaller group – not everyone – who gets stuck in a cycle of pain?

'And lots of people who have chronic back pain, they can't even pinpoint a moment when it started,' says Maher. 'The back is incredibly well-designed and incredibly strong.'

Really, I'm not sure what the answer is – but I do think the point is a bit moot. This is our spine. We can't evolve past it. We have to live with it – and work out how to stop it hurting. 'Horses walk around on four legs and still get back pain – so do dachshunds,' says Maher. 'It's not to do with two legs. And if it was, what are we going to tell people to do? Walk around on their arms?'

2   You can't slip a disc

After viewing McMenamin's spines, I decided I would start with the most obvious 'weak' spot: the disc. In the modern history of back pain, there is no more maligned body part. We have blamed it, tested it, punctured it, injected it, used radiation to melt parts of it, and then, when all that has failed, we've cut it out. It is seen as a tiny cause of enormous misery. For many, a black disc on a scan is like a death sentence for the spine.

I should know. When I was about 17, one of my discs slipped. I knew as soon as it went. I leaned my weight forward onto the wheeled cage laden with crates of tinned tuna I was pushing, bent my back, and felt a sharp jab of pain on the right side of my spine, just above my hip, as though I'd been stabbed with a ballpoint pen. My entire back seized. The burning enveloped my lower back and quickly ran all the way up the long muscles that run alongside my spine. I stopped hard, and the cage slid gently away down the floodlit supermarket aisle. I knew what I'd done. I reached back with one hand, and I swear I could feel the protruding surface sticking hard into the muscle. Sweating and almost giddy with adrenaline and endorphins, I wandered through empty aisles to find my manager, shook my head at him. I was done.

Just like my dad.

At home, I spent the next week copying everything my dad did to deal with back pain. I lay on Mum's red foam yoga mat, my back flat, my head propped up to watch television, as the hard floor pushed my discs back into position. I refused to lift anything heavy, in fear I would worsen the damage. My boss at the supermarket approved my request to switch onto check-out duty, relieved, I guess, that I hadn't thought of making a WorkCover claim.

After that, I carried it around for years. 'Slipped disc,' I told people, 'L4.' Or L5, maybe. Dad's physio soon confirmed my own diagnosis. He liked to strap me up to a traction table, which would slowly, by means of a winch, pull my legs away from my hips. 'This will open up the spaces between your vertebrae, give your discs a chance to breathe', he explained, and I nodded, as though I were a veteran of all this; as though Dad's experiences had been my own.

And Dad's story *was* the same as mine, at least in outline. He'd always told me he hurt his back when he was young. But stories seemed to change, or slip, or maybe I'm remembering them wrong. There was an accident playing basketball – he landed too heavily and slipped a disc? I called Dad, and this time he told a new story.

His mother, my grandmother – a terrifying Norwegian immigrant – decided to relocate her small family to Coward Springs, deep in the desert country of South Australia. With no one else to help her, Dad ended up the designated labourer, at age 14, chopping jarrah sleepers for firewood with an increasingly blunt axe; carrying 20-litre jerrycans of water from the bore; lugging jerrycans of fuel to pour – by hand – into the vehicles of travellers who stopped to buy at the store, and using tyre levers and heavy steel bead-breakers to change tyres. Dad said his surgeon told him that probably damaged his back for life. 'He basically told me that I'd done what school kids are told not to do – carry heavy weights while the discs in the back are forming,' he said.

From the moment of diagnosis by Dad's physio, every bit of back pain I experienced was explained by that disc, and I carried the pain with me everywhere I went. If I took a particularly hard step in hard-soled business shoes, or jumped from the bus onto the pavement, I felt the vibrations right there in my damaged disc. I felt it swell in anger and pain and shrink again after a couple of ibuprofen. I felt it pretty much right up to the time James McAuley looked at me in rising fury.

'A slipped disc?' he said, eyes wild. 'That makes absolutely no sense at all. It's impossible. You can't slip a disc. It does not exist.'

Listening back to my recorded interview with him, I cringe a little. Half my questions are little more than an incredulous '*Really?*'

Like when McAuley says something like: 'Everyone has disc bulges. Even things like disc prolapse, people without back pain have some evidence of that.'

'*Really?*'

You know how, just like every cheap motel room looks the same, GPs' offices have a *look*? Almost as though there's a big department store they all shop at, a medical IKEA. Cheap and uncomfortable plastic chairs, big examination bed upholstered in squeaky vinyl, reading chart on the wall, deflated blood pressure cuff, and a big white model of the spine. Why every GP needs their own miniature spine, I'm not sure, but it's nearly always there.

The bones are a bleached white plastic, and the vertebrae are separated from each other by yellow discs. Sandwiched in there between the bones, the discs look thin and vulnerable, like they're liable to just slip right out at any time.

James McAuley really, really hates that spine.

'Discs don't look like that!' McAuley exclaims, wide-eyed, fury curdling in this mild-mannered professor. 'They look nothing like that. They are these really hard things that join the spine together.' He holds that model spine almost singularly responsible for the idea of 'slipped discs'. Which, he says, aren't a real thing.

When I was struggling with my 'slipped disc', I imagined it a bit like a loose Jenga block, and my spine was the unstable Jenga tower. The block – my disc – edged out and jabbed me. But that's not how discs look or work at all.

Spinal discs are like jam doughnuts: a hard shell filled with jelly. Were you to slide one of your discs out of your spine and cup it in your hand, it would be about the size of a 50 cent coin. You have 23, sandwiched between the vertebrae of the neck (cervical), chest (thoracic) and lower back (lumbar). (The vertebrae of the lower parts of the spine – the sacrum and coccyx – are fused.)

The disc gives you flexibility and shock absorption. Imagine a spine where the bony vertebrae were just rubbing on each other; there would be no bend and every footfall would reverberate right up into your skull.

For something so crucial, the discs are almost totally devoid of blood flow. Oxygen and nutrients must reach the disc from blood vessels that run down the very edges of the structure. The outer parts of the disc are supposed to ferry those essential chemicals into the gooey centre, which has no blood supply of its own.

That makes the centre of the disc a place pretty unlike the rest of your body. With little oxygen available, the cells rely on anaerobic respiration – they almost don't need oxygen to live. That process generates lactic acid, which means your disc is essentially living in an acidic stew with almost no oxygen or nutrients. Not that it minds. It has adapted extraordinarily well. The cells are so hardy, they go on living happily for hours – even days – after a person dies. Two days after you or I shuffle off this mortal coil, says Professor Chris Little, head of a bone and joint research lab at the University of Sydney, surgeons could still extract living cells from our discs.

A small chunk of gel the size of a 50-cent piece, with no oxygen to breathe, barely any blood supply or nutrients, and a whole spine to hold up. No wonder, you might think, the disc gets sore. 'It's a precarious environment,' says Chris Little.

But discs are designed to be hardy. They're the body's shock distributors. And they rarely complain. They can't, by design, as they barely have any nerve endings. There are some nerves on the outside of the disc, but in a healthy spine, they don't go any further than 3 millimetres deep.[1] The entire inner centre of the disc, nearly all its volume, is totally without feeling.

Unlike hard bone, the disc is designed to move and change as you do different things during the day; as more or less pressure is put through it, it is supposed to flatten and bulge. During the day, the discs are slowly squished down as you stand upright, losing 25 per cent of their thickness.

They regain this at night, swelling with water and nutrients as you lie in bed. Lift heavy weights at the gym and they'll also shrink slightly – by about 3.6 millimetres across the entire spine, according to one small study.[2]

And they don't look anything like the thin yellow plastic discs in those desktop models.

When a surgeon removes a disc, it is not a matter of simply opening up the space and sliding out the disc like a hamburger. The discs are firmly attached to the spine. They cannot slip out to either side.

'The term "slipped disc" is just not accurate,' says Professor Mark Hancock, a leading back pain researcher at Macquarie University. 'It physically can't. The disc is extremely strongly attached to the vertebrae above and below.'

Your disc can't slide out. However, several things can go wrong with it. First, the disc can *herniate* – the hard outer ring can fracture or puncture, squeezing some of its jelly-like filling out. This can put pressure on a nearby nerve, causing sciatica – pain down the leg. We often call this 'slipping a disc', but as you can see, it doesn't really resemble a slip.

Lesley Podesta was in the middle of a holiday in Vietnam when she grasped the handles of a heavy suitcase – too heavy – twisted and yanked. Pop. Instant blinding pain. 'I am very, very good with pain,' she tells me. 'And I felt like there was glass scraping on bone all down my leg and through my pelvis. It was unrelenting. It was terrible.'

Podesta had just herniated a disc in her lower back. The disc's goo, ejected under high pressure, crushed the nerves that ran down into her legs. For months, she could barely walk, managing only a bent-backed shuffle. Her doctor put her on the heavy-duty anti-inflammatory prednisolone. It barely helped. Her surgeon offered her a laminectomy – a decompression surgery to take pressure off the spinal nerves.

It must have been tempting. But Lesley isn't for quick fixes. 'I'd heard too many stories, and I wanted to see if there was another option first before going for surgery,' she says. 'I knew if I could get through the intense pain, I could probably learn to manage things.'

She opted for the conservative course: physiotherapy, psychology and careful and diligent gym work to rebuild her strength, allowing her muscles to take pressure off her spine. 'I've really focused on building up my strength, so I feel less fragile. Physiotherapy has been really good. What I had not appreciated was how important it was to strengthen all the other muscles, and change some of the ways I moved,' she says.

It's taken a while, but she's pleased with her progress and is now largely pain-free. Her body, which felt like it was failing her, no longer holds her back. She is strong. I ask her if she has any advice for other people with back pain. She thinks for a moment. 'You should get expert support, and not self-diagnose,' she says. 'People who've been educated and trained are your best friends. Don't pretend you can work it out on the internet. Partner with someone who's going to look after your back, strengthen it. And it's no crime to need pain relief.'

The difference between sciatica and back pain

The sciatic nerve is the largest nerve in the body.[3] It runs from the lower part of your back, through your buttocks and down your legs, dividing into smaller branches as it goes. Squeeze it – say via a herniated disc – and you get pain down the leg, and maybe muscle weakness or tingling. Material squeezed out of the disc can also cause an inflammatory response in the nerve, turning it red and swollen. Doctors will often test for sciatica by asking you to lie on the bed before they slowly raise your painful leg in the air, stretching the tender nerve. If you shriek and curse, you've possibly got sciatica.

'These nerves come out of the spine. If they get compressed, they may cause leg pain, which can range from mild to severe,' spine surgeon Dr Michael Johnson tells me, tracing the thick nerves with his finger across the laptop screen.

'But only leg pain?'

'No,' says Johnson, 'the symptoms can be variable. The predominant symptom is usually leg pain, but there may be a component of back pain.

'Now if you relieve the compression by removing the prolapse, the leg pain will be improved. This is called sciatica – and it's quite different to back pain.'

This is important for our story, so let's spell it out. Sciatica is commonly caused by a herniated disc. The key symptom is leg pain, not back pain. *Plenty of people have disc bulges and signs of damage without any back pain.* It takes a fair amount of nerve compression to produce pain. A disc bulge and other minor deformities are generally not enough. This explains why sciatica is not common.

While there are many bad treatments for back pain, treatment for sciatica is a shining light. While sciatica will settle naturally for about 90 per cent of people, if you still have acute pain, surgery can provide effective rapid relief.[4]

'We're very good at helping people who have nerves injured, strangled, compressed,' says Brisbane-based neurosurgeon Associate Professor Sarah Olsen. 'We're not very good at helping mechanical back pain.'

'The cause of a person's back pain is often more difficult to identify – so surgery is more unreliable and less frequently appropriate,' says Dr Johnson.

It is the blurring of sciatica and back pain that has led to many people undergoing operations that are unsuccessful, and which may make things worse.

'So,' I say to Dr Johnson, thinking out loud, 'my dad never had leg pain. For it to be sciatica, do you have to have leg pain?'

'No, not always,' said Dr Johnson. 'Sometimes it's just buttock pain. Sometimes – unusually – it can be just back pain. And the people that spine surgery can most reliably assist are people with pain due to nerve compression. Surgery for back pain is only occasionally appropriate.'

Gary Collins (not his real name) spent years struggling with severe pain in his lower back, hips and thighs – caused by a compressed sciatic nerve, he was told. Rather than having a decompression, his surgeon opted for a fusion – a surgery with an extremely dubious evidence base, as we will explore in Chapter 9.

At Collins's first consult with the surgeon, he was told his chances of being pain-free post surgery were better than 90 per cent. Five months after the surgery, Collins was much worse – his pain was intense and he could barely move. The same surgeon opened up his spine again, but the pain did not improve.

The surgeon charged Collins through the nose, including thousands of dollars that his private insurance did not cover, all to be paid up front. After the surgery, the surgeon who had assured Collins of success did not want a bar of him – Collins was left in the care of nurses. He now won't return Collins's emails or phone calls.

'He doesn't know what's causing the pain as the procedures are OK,' says Collins. 'He suggested I make an appointment with a neurologist.'

Collins got in touch after reading an article I wrote about fusion's poor success rates. After browsing though several studies, he could see none of them even came close to the surgeon's '90-per-cent-plus' claim. 'He's a charlatan and in it for the money only,' Collins says. 'He should be reported to the authorities and deregistered.'

But you don't always have to have surgery to recover from nerve compression. 'Large numbers of people with nerve compression get better by themselves,' says Dr Johnson.

'What?' I say. 'The disc …'

'Resorbs spontaneously,' Dr Johnson says, nodding. He pulls up another slide, a spinal MRI showing a prolapsed disc. 'Here's a disc prolapse there. This is with no treatment. And then three months later …'

'Oh,' I say. It was gone.

How could a prolapsed disc just slide back in? It was like a Jenga tower spontaneously rebuilding itself, a magic trick. Scientists are still a bit puzzled by this phenomenon, and don't really understand how it works, nor what prompts a ruptured disc to pack itself up again, and why this does not happen in all cases. But they know it happens. In one case study of 42 people with herniated discs, 88 per cent of them had seen their discs substantially heal – by themselves – within 12 months.[5] Their back pain had improved in step with this healing. A systematic review published in 2015 found that 70 per cent of extruded discs naturally healed on their own. Indeed, the more of the disc that had herniated, the more *likely* it was to heal.[6]

Part of the problem, I think, is that we live in a mechanical world and like to think of our bodies as machines made up of individual components: heart and lungs and spine and discs. If the machine breaks down, just swap out the faulty part and you're on your way. This works in some cases – hip replacements or kidney transplants – but humans are ultimately not machines. We're large creatures made up of billions of individual cells, inhabited by billions more bacterial cells that live in harmony with us. We aren't built piece by piece but rather grow from an egg – and we can adapt and repair.

That takes us back to one of the core themes that seemed to repeat as I read more papers and spoke to more scientists: the body is nothing, *nothing* like a car. Cars are made of hard components that push up against each other and fracture under the strain. Our bodies, by contrast, are made of soft, living components that grow stronger under strain. And they can heal themselves, if we give them the chance. The more you learn about how disc herniation works, the less and less the term 'slipped disc' makes any sense.

I called Dad later that evening, keen to pick over Dr Johnson's MRIs. It sounded like the surgeon had solved Dad's issue. It was sciatica.

But that wasn't right, Dad insisted. He'd never had weakness or pain in his leg. Or in his butt. And the pain he did have, in his back, flared sporadically, rather than sticking around stubbornly. 'And if your nerve is being compressed, shouldn't you have pain all the time? And I didn't have that,' he said.

'The surgeon never offered to fix my sciatica. He said he'd fix the disc bulges. When I asked him why there was no sciatic nerve problem, he said "That happens sometimes",' Dad says.

3 Disc degeneration – not a problem?

Dad introduced me to the gym. 'A strong body and a strong core,' he told me. 'You need both.' It would become the habit of a lifetime. When we first started going together, Dad's back was sore but he was still holding it together. The gym was central to his plans. He'd build a strong back and core; he'd exercise his way out of pain.

I remember standing, waiting for a turn on a weight machine, watching the serious weightlifters work. They'd grasp a barbell in one hand, hang it down to the side, and then bend down with it, lowering the weight to their knee, before pulling their spine back upright. Dad was horrified. A recipe for disc damage, he told me – just as his physiotherapist had told him. Every degree the spine bent added 10 kilos of pressure to each disc … or something. Every time you lifted with a flexed back you risked blowing out a disc. I remember feeling distinctly sorry for those large men, doomed to a lifetime of back failure as they aged.

Your lifestyle is likely not hurting your back

It's 'common knowledge' that our lifestyles can put our discs at risk. There's an entire section of the wellness industry engaged in keeping your discs healthy. Improve your posture. Lift with a straight back. Sleep on a firm mattress. Drink lots of water. Scientists have been equally worried. Back in the 1990s they fretted over the damage heavy lifting or the vibrations from long-distance truck driving might be doing to our discs. So in 1991 team of researchers recruited hundreds of twins across Finland and bussed them in for an intensive two-day physical and mental investigation.[1] Blood, DNA and urine tests were done. Back muscles were checked for thickness and power. Diet, smoking, exercise levels, back pain and job history were collected and catalogued. Each twin was asked to work out how much weight they lifted in their job, how often, and how long they spent sitting. And an MRI was done of each and every twin's spine.

In his office Dr Michael Johnson shows me the study's results. 'These are two different twins,' he says, pulling the MRI up on his laptop. 'One's a computer engineer and the other's a plumber. And you can see the MRIs are almost identical. Here's another one. One's a farmer, the other's a chauffeur.'

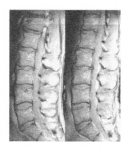 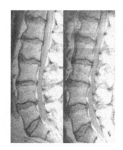

Programmer / Plumber (48 years old)   Farmer / Chauffeur (61 years old)

I looked closely. You could barely tell the difference. There was certainly no evidence an occupation that put extra stress and strain on your back wore out your discs and verte-brae any faster. As the scientists behind the study wrote, they could not find a single thing in a person's environment that seemed to put them at greater risk of disc degeneration. What a person did in life, how they lived, their posture, how much load they put through their discs – all that had only a tiny, tiny effect on disc degeneration.

'In fact,' wrote the surprised scientists, 'some indications were found that routine loading may actually have some benefits to the disc.' Other work since has furthered this suspicion.

The study, and later ones, suggested genes play a much larger role in how a person's discs degenerate. And there's little we can do about them.

But like many parts of back pain, what scientists know is a long way from what the public believe. How many times have you heard someone warn you against wearing your body out? This mindset – that our bodies degrade if we push them – holds many back from physical exercise of the type that has been shown to improve our physical and mental health in many ways, and leaves some back pain sufferers fearing that they're trapped in a slow physical decline, cursed to get worse and worse until they end up in a wheelchair.

Disc bulges and degeneration do not necessarily cause pain

So ... we can't do much about our discs growing old. It's in our genes. How much of a *problem* is a dodgy disc?

Dr Johnson furrows his brow and flicks through the images on his laptop, before finally pulling an image up on his screen – a black and white MRI, the scan taken from side on, showing the bones of the spine in white, the discs in grey, and the surrounding flesh in black.

'This is actually my daughter,' he says. 'I'm sure she won't mind. So this was when she was in … year 11, I think.'

She'd been complaining of a sore back. Surprisingly common among kids, Dr Johnson says. So they'd MRI'd her.

His fingers trace the line of her spine. Healthy discs all the way down, until we get to the problem area. Two thin, black discs, that look to be offering all the support of soggy cardboard. Degeneration. If I saw that on my scan, I'd be flipping out.

What do you do when you're a top spinal surgeon and your daughter has a degenerating spine? Physio? A remedial exercise program? Surgery?

The answer turns out to be 'none of the above'. You do nothing.

'I haven't heard her complain for three or four years,' says Dr Johnson. 'And she's very active, goes to the gym, plays basketball, runs. There's just not a very strong correlation between disc degeneration and back pain.'

Disc degeneration, Dr Johnson tells me, isn't a symptom of a crumbling spine. It happens in young and old and, for the vast majority of people, causes no pain or disability – no symptoms at all. Scan me or you, your children or even Dr Johnson and you'll probably find a disc that looks degenerate. We all have them. They're normal, says Dr Johnson. They seem to wear out at their own pace; there's not much we can do to speed it up or slow it down. And most of the time they don't cause us any problems. They'll usually heal up fine.

What happened to Dr Johnson's daughter? Likely, her discs healed and resumed their work in the spine. Or maybe they didn't heal – and she'll be fine with that too.

This may shock you. It certainly shocks me. It is a scientific finding that has not yet permeated the general community, perhaps because it doesn't make intuitive sense. X-rays show bone clean and white against dark tissue. White, strong and healthy. *Of course* that blackened sliver that used to be your disc is causing your back pain. But the published scientific evidence, Dr Johnson points out, simply does not support that idea.

In 2015 the *American Journal of Neuroradiology* published what is now a highly cited systematic review of the evidence for spinal degeneration in people *without* back pain.[2] Scientists really like systematic reviews. They are put together by teams of researchers who spend months or years trying to find every relevant study on a specific topic. By putting all the results of the smaller studies together, you get a really powerful piece of evidence you can trust more than a small single study.[3] The 2015 review gathered together 33 smaller studies covering 3110 people *without* back pain. In each of these studies, scientists had CT'd or MRI'd the spine, looking for signs of health or decay. You think a decaying spine is rare, or bad? That's not what the numbers say. Almost a third of the 20 year olds had a disc bulge. Some 37 per cent of 20 year olds had clear signs of disc degeneration. That rose to 96 per cent in people aged 80. To repeat: these were people *without back pain.*

Think about what this means. It means millions of people are walking around right now with disc bulges or degeneration and *no pain at all.*

One clinical pain textbook notes MRI studies in people without back pain have found herniated discs in up to 70 per cent of people, degeneration in up to 50 per cent, and tears in the disc in up to 20 per cent.[4] But these studies have repeatedly failed to show those structural problems are going to *cause* back pain, or even make it particularly more likely.

That's the best evidence. Personally I think the *most compelling* comes from a study done at the Richmond marathon in London, a 42-kilometre race which winds through Kew Gardens and down the Thames.[5] A group of 28 runners were recruited in 2019 for a study; none had ever run a marathon and none had back pain. They all underwent an MRI and then spent four months training for the race, and then, after crossing the finish line, went in for another MRI. At the first scan, 17 had signs of disc degeneration – more than half the group, despite *no one* having back pain. And after going through four months of hard training and then pounding the pavement over the course of the marathon, the follow-up MRI revealed no signs of any increased damage. That gives me a lot of confidence: even if my discs are bad, that's no guarantee I'll get back pain – and nothing I do is going to make them worse.

One of the study's authors, Professor Alister Hart, a hip surgeon who sees many patients with back pain and who holds the chair of orthopaedics at London's Royal National Orthopaedic Hospital, told me he found the results a real surprise.

'The take-home [message] is that the MRI appearance of our discs should not put us off from running,' he says. 'Running strengthens the muscles that support the spine which maintains alignment and more evenly spreads the load on the discs.'

Indeed, far from wearing your discs down, running may actually be *good* for them. In the last few years research has started to emerge showing that people who run a lot have more-hydrated, thicker, healthier discs; the same thing is seen in animals.[6] 'It's similar to how lifting heavy weights stimulates our muscles to become bigger and stronger, and jumping and bounding can make our bones more dense and less prone to fracture,' says Patrick Owen.

Disc degeneration seems to start almost at birth. In 2003 a researcher presented MRI scans of the discs of 154 ten-year-old children, looking for signs of disc degeneration.[7] The scans were reviewed by two independent clinicians. In 9 per cent of the children, they found clear signs of disc degeneration. It was a finding that drew worldwide headlines. Our spines were starting to fail us before we graduated high school! And here were the poor bubs, the innocent condemned to a life of back pain. One website illustrated its coverage with a picture of a pained young child, lying in bed next to his toy rabbit. 'Some kids may be set up for a lifetime of low back pain,' the caption read.

But if they were condemned, the kids did not know it yet. When asked, none of the kids with dodgy discs said they had back pain.

'You can look at a group of patients and they might all have changes – but their pain would be totally different, ranging from no pain to very high pain,' says Dr Hazel Jenkins, a Macquarie University researcher who studies spine scans and back pain. Why? That, Dr Jenkins says, remains one of the great mysteries of back pain. We don't know. 'For a lot of the things we see on the X-ray, there is just not good evidence for how they might be affecting the patient. And it's very unclear whether the changes are related to the pain or not.'

Nor were these children any more likely to go on to have a sore back. In a long-term study, young men with signs of disc degeneration at age 20 were no more likely to report back pain over the next 30 years than those who had healthy-looking discs.[8]

Part of the problem with the disc, some scientists now think, may not be physical at all. It's the words we use to describe it. Bulging. Herniated. *Degenerated.*

When things go wrong with the disc, those words make it sound like they go really, spectacularly wrong – like you're degenerating and falling apart – when really, often all they're describing is the natural – and harmless – march of aging. We don't call hair turning grey 'hair degeneration'. 'We think of degeneration as being a bad thing,' says Associate Professor Paige Little, an expert on discs at the Queensland University of Technology. 'I don't think it is. As you get older, you don't necessarily want to have the same amount of motion as you did when you were young. I don't think you want to be bending, stretching and turning as much when you get to 50 or 60 as you did when you were 20 or 25. Maybe that's the body's natural way of saying "slow down a bit, I want you to last a bit longer".'

How the disc was cast as villain

The key to thinking about the disc, says back pain researcher Chris Maher, is this: 'The current guidelines suggest that for the bulk of people, clinicians cannot reliably say what structure is the cause of your back pain.'

How, then, did we start believing all back pain was caused by small lumps within our spine that we can't see? How did the way we think about our discs get so out of sync with the evidence?

The answer may be a simple medical mistake made long ago.

For the vast stretch of human history our ancestors gave no thought to their discs – because they didn't know they were there. The Greeks' medical texts barely mention back pain, while the Romans thought it was caused by disturbed humours.[9] In the Middle Ages, the Germans blamed witches for back pain (the modern German word for low back pain, *hexenschuss*, literally means 'witch's shot'), while the Welsh blamed elves. As late as the 17th century, physicians were blaming cold damp weather for back pain.[10]

Up until this point no one had ever really blamed the *spine* for back pain. Back pain was caused by something external, something that happened to you, rather than a creeping degradation. And it wasn't taken too seriously. It was just a fact of life.

That changed in 1828, thanks to Thomas Brown. Dr Brown, a senior physician at Glasgow's Royal Infirmary, took an interest in a Miss C, aged 17 – her name sadly lost to history.[11] The young woman was hale and healthy, except for a spot of back pain that refused to go away. A 'gnawed, bruised' feeling that got worse when she was tired, better when she lay down, and wasn't sore to the touch. She'd had all the standard treatments: bleeding, blistering. Her pain refused to improve.

Brown ran his hand along the vertebrae of her spine, pushing at each level. As he neared the midpoint of her ribcage, Miss C gave a startled yelp. There was the pain, shooting through her back from the place where Brown's fingers were. She hadn't even known her spine was sore. So different was society's attitude to back pain at the time, it seems, she hadn't even thought to check.

The physician sent her for a dose of ten leeches at the site, to suck out the inflammation. She made a full recovery, Brown noted in an essay for the *Glasgow Medical Journal*. He called Miss C's problem 'spinal irritation' – a disorder, he thought, of the nerves that run through the spine, referring pain to other places in the body.

Brown's little pamphlet swept the US and Europe, attracting attention from leading doctors around the world.[12] Brown's idea was never proven, and gradually disappeared. But it changed the back pain game because it linked pain with a damaged spine. This was an important leap. Brown noted the spinal nerves were the problem, but he didn't call it 'irritated nerves', but 'spinal irritation' – as though the spine itself were at fault. And there was no putting that idea back in the bottle.

Barely 32 years later, Britain was gripped by a panic, something like an Industrial Revolution version of the Y2K bug. Men and women exposed to the violent jostling of the shiny new steam trains which were suddenly replacing horses and carts across the nation were reporting mysterious symptoms: exhaustion, trembling, paralysis, chronic pain. It was clear to the doctors of the time that all the jostling and shaking of rail travel was doing something terrible to the spines of train passengers. 'Railway spine', they called it, and it was considered a very serious disorder – people could recover, but they would never be the same.[13]

Railway spine is, thankfully, no longer widely diagnosed. But look at the way the thinking about back pain had changed in a short space of years: from being overlooked and ignored, to being viewed as a minor problem caused by something external, to then being seen as a life-threatening condition caused by some internal disfigurement or injury – and it did not even have to be a bad injury – centred on the spine.

But it was in the New World that the disc finally claimed its modern role as villain-in-chief.

William Jason Mixter, a prominent Boston neuro-surgeon once described as 'the man in New England who knew the most about the spine', and Joseph S Barr, a young and ambitious orthopaedic surgeon, met in the corridor outside a patient's room in the Bullfinch building at Massachusetts General Hospital.[14] It was the spring of 1932. Inside, lying in bed, was a young man with a very bad back.

KN had come off his skis two years earlier, smashing his lower back. The pain flowed like live electric wire from his back down his left side and into his calf. He'd spent two years receiving standard treatment for the injury, including a long period totally immobilised inside a frame. The pain was no better.

Mixter had been asked to open KN up and see what was going wrong. Digging with his scalpel, he found what looked like a large tumour pressing on the man's spinal nerves. After removing it, the man's symptoms went away. It seemed like yet another success for a brilliant surgeon.

But Barr wasn't convinced. Other tests for spinal tumours had come back negative. Why would he suddenly develop a tumour? Why would one sprout at the exact time he was falling off his skis? What if, he said to Mixter, the man's pain came from a dislodged disc, rather than a tumour?

The pair decided to investigate. They collected samples from all the 'tumours' that were being taken out of patients' spines at the hospital. Sure enough, they reported in a paper published in 1934, the tissue wasn't tumour at all. It was ruptured disc material. Sciatica – back pain that radiates down into the leg and foot – was being caused not by tumours growing in the spine but by a damaged disc pushing out into the path of the nerves. Remove the pressure and you can pretty reliably cure the pain.

Mixter and Barr's contribution was to recognise that what had previously been called chondromas – tumours – were actually fragments of the intervertebral disc, one of Mixter's biographers, New Hampshire–based neurosurgeon Dr Perry Ball, tells me. 'Even today, the large majority of cases of sciatica are due to disc herniation – so this was an important insight in terms of understanding the cause of a common symptom.'

The paper took the world by storm. It changed sciatica treatment from a conservative approach to one requiring surgery – although Mixter and Barr's contemporaries had to overlook the fact that at least four of the patients in the original paper died and two had complete paraplegia.[15]

Nevertheless, this triumphant moment is one of those instances history hinges on. If we stop the tape here, Mixter and Barr's spots in the spinal surgery hall of fame are uncontested.

A year later, Mixter – by this time no longer working with Barr – published a new and much more radical paper that made several key contributions that would shape back pain for decades to come.[16]

First, the paper coined the term 'herniation or rupture of the intervertebral disc' rather than the less scary sounding 'prolapse of the nucleus pulposus'. Second, it linked that with trauma or injury to the spine – despite several patients *insisting* they'd never injured their back or discs.[17] (We now know minor injuries aren't more likely to lead to serious low back pain, even in people with pre-existing structural changes to the spine.[18])

Most importantly, Mixter wrote that a ruptured disc could cause back pain *without any sign of nerve involvement*. Cutting it out could cure it – a claim that seemed to ignore the fact that several patients ended up with a 'lame back' after the operation (and one died).[19]

This is the key: a bulging disc did more than cause sciatica by pinching nerves in the back, the surgeon claimed. *It also caused back pain.* Mixter's paper opened the way for a new view: disc bulging was not a natural part of aging but bad, and a cause of back pain – oh, and it was fixable via surgery.

Right there you have the birth of modern back pain medicine. The disc is the source of back pain, and we can and *must* cut it out. The 'dynasty of the disc', some textbooks call it. 'The disc was thereafter made responsible for all kinds of back and leg pain – and many treatments were the consequence,' note Philipp Gruber and Thomas Boeni in a classic textbook.

From an ignored lump of bone, within a decade the disc had become the site and cause of 90 per cent of all back pain.[20] It 'unleashed on the unsuspecting public a wave of surgical enthusiasm', writes Gordon Waddell.[21] In scientific journals, other theories of back pain almost completely disappear as the disc takes centre stage.[22] Before Mixter and Barr's discovery, back pain treatment tended to be conservative; after the discovery, it became the domain of the surgeon.

The disc became such a popular back pain villain it was labelled a 'diagnosis of exclusion': if nothing else fits, it's probably disc pain.[23] 'If the disc is the evil pain generator, removing the disc should be curative,' writes Dr Nortin Hadler in his book on the back pain medico-industry, *Stabbed in the Back*. 'Questioning the credo was heresy, and to a large extent is heresy still.' Surgeons started, tentatively, by making a diagnosis based on hard evidence of nerve problems; those evidence requirements were soon watered down.[24] But still, they knew a lot of people had disc problems – you could see them on the damn scan – and there were a lot of people with back pain. It became as simple as putting two and two together and getting disc surgery.

This credo also happened to make everyone a lot of money. At one time, it was claimed the average American neurosurgeon made half his income from disc surgery.[25]

But even in those exciting early days, there were obvious problems. It was widely accepted that 90 per cent of back pain was caused by the disc, but when surgeons opened up a patient they often found, to their disappointment, no obvious disc problems. Doubters were starting to claim that many of the positive findings in surgery were lies being told to cover up a surgeon's rash decision to operate.[26]

In 1941, a clever Baltimore surgeon by the name of Walter Dandy came up with a solution that solved all these problems: the concealed disc. In some cases, he proposed, the disc bulge was so small it was discernible only by careful surgical inspection – it felt 'distinctly softer to the touch than a normal disc,' he wrote. But it was there. Rather than being overemphasised, Dandy wrote, we were just 'scratching the surface' of the disc's contribution to back pain.

If a patient complained of long-lasting back and leg pain, made worse by sneezing, the surgeon could be confident of a disc problem. So confident, urged Dandy, they did not even need to bother with diagnostic tests.

These men were acting with the best of intentions (and also were making a lot of money), but they did tremendous damage to our understanding of the back. Damage we are still trying to undo now. '[Disc surgery] was accused of leaving more tragic human wreckage in its wake than any other operation in history,' writes Waddell.

Later in his life, Joseph Barr had some regrets. He authored a psychological study of 36 patients with back pain.[27] In 14 cases, he admitted, no physical problems could be found, and yet those patients consistently reported life-destroying chronic pain. The man who had invented the evocative and terrifying term 'ruptured disc' had come to regret he ever coined it due to the obvious psychological damage the phrase was doing, writes Hadler.[28]

Today, the role of the disc in back pain remains deeply controversial. 'It's still an enigma. We don't know all the answers yet. And there is a frustration there, because we've been trying to understand back pain for so long,' says Dr Paige Little, an expert on the disc based at the University of Queensland.

We now know that a degenerated, damaged or herniated disc is no guarantee of back pain, as was once thought. And we know the vast majority of people with back pain won't have any evidence on a scan of anything physical being wrong.[29] But discs do play a role.

The disc can herniate. It can degrade. It can tear. It can stop properly distributing load across the spine. It can impinge on nerves other than the ones that cause sciatica. All these things can be the cause of back pain. And while most people with disc degeneration do not have symptoms, having a degenerated disc makes you about twice as likely to have back pain, the best evidence we have suggests.[30]

When a disc is damaged, small tears appear on its surface. This is how the 'jelly' inside the disc escapes into the spinal canal. The body is capable of healing the disc. But as the inflammation goes to work, rebuilding the disc, it may also rebuild new nerves inside the torn surface of the disc.[31] These new nerves may be important for healing, but they are certainly not supposed to be there.

'That means each time you do something, bend, twist, turn in bed, the nerves in the disc are recording some pressure. And they send a signal to the muscles around, and that creates muscle spasm and pain,' one spinal surgeon told me. A damaged disc may also leak nutrients and inflammatory cells, causing pain.

But, as we've seen, many people have disc herniation or degradation and *no* back pain.

Consider this study: in 2017, researchers in Holland were running a large, high-quality trial of radiofrequency denervation – essentially, hot wires are used to burn off any nerve causing pain, often near an allegedly painful disc.[32] If nerves going into the disc were causing the pain, burning them off should stop that pain. 'They go round the disc, they fry the nerve endings. They're gone. It can't produce pain,' says Professor James McAuley. And yet, the subjects did not experience less pain; researchers were unable to find any improvement in pain scores. Burning the nerves made no difference. 'And to me, that says pain is more complex than what's happening in the disc,' says McAuley. 'It absolutely has to be.'

Discograms and spinal fusions

Discs can play a role in back pain. But here's the problem: short of cutting them out, we have no way of knowing which discs have nerves growing into them. Scans cannot tell a painful disc from a pain-free one.[33] And the technique surgeons often turn to to prove which disc is the cause of pain – discograms – have serious flaws.

'Despite what you've been told, the discogram is not designed to create agony,' the website of one pain clinic cheerfully notes. To run a discogram, also known as discography, a doctor inserts thin needles through the skin and into the discs. A small amount of dye is squirted down the needle, increasing pressure inside the disc, simulating the pressure discs encounter when you're walking around. In theory, when the damaged disc is subject to those pressures it will kick off the back pain.

As the surgeon works their way up or down the spine, your job is to yell out when you feel pressure or pain. 'It was horrible,' wrote one woman on an Australian spinal fusion support group. They injected her in two discs; the lower one produced only a small amount of pain, but when they did the upper it produced pain that was 'horrible, sharp … right up my spinal cord'.

'They had three unsuccessful tries,' wrote another woman online. 'Pain radiated down my leg. I just wanted to jump off the bed! I had no pain with [the] successful needle, but pain got intense throughout the day and the next. What does that say?'

A successful discography diagnosis often leads to a spinal fusion to fix disc pain.[34] And if discography worked reliably, this suffering would be worth it and back pain medicine would be so much simpler. We could simply pick out the damaged disc and fix it.

Alas, it does not.

Amazingly, it took many decades from the procedure's invention for a serious study on the effectiveness of discography to be done. Dr Eugene Carragee, an orthopaedic surgeon at the Stanford University School of Medicine, tracked 25 people with back pain over five years.[35] Each was given a discogram at the start of the trial. In the people who tested positive for disc problems – 12 in Carragee's study – the expectation was that nearly all would go on to develop back pain. But this did not happen. Even the people who reported the most pain from the discogram were no more likely to end up with long-term back problems.

Carragee followed this up with a second study in 2009, tracking 30 patients who had positive discograms and underwent spinal fusion. Just eight had good outcomes from the surgery; less than half even had what the surgeon defined as a 'minimal accepted outcome'.

The problem seems to be this: discography is really, really painful, whether you have an injured disc or not. It's easy for a surgeon – or a desperate patient – to misidentify the pain as meaning the disc is damaged.

'The evidence strongly suggests that pain with disc injection is a non-specific phenomenon, often unrelated to the cause of a low back pain syndrome,' Carragee would later write. Despite 60 years of research, he wrote, no one had ever proven it useful for caring for people with low back pain.

The worst was to come when Carragee presented his findings at the International Society for the Study of the Lumbar Spine annual meeting in Miami in 2009, including a new study that suggested all that jabbing, puncturing and injecting of the disc with a needle might actually accelerate disc degradation.[36] Not only did the test not work, it made things worse. Carragee had been following a group of patients with serious low back pain for ten years; 52 had received discographies to diagnose back pain and 50 had not. Over the next decade, the spinal discs of those who had been jabbed degraded significantly more, lost more height, and were at more risk of herniation than those who had not had the procedure, often on the side where the disc had been punctured.

'Well,' remarked Gordon Brown, a doctor based at the University of Miami, 'you've just killed off discography. In the face of your findings, and the fact that discography has no utility, I think we will have to inform our patients that there is a problem. I think you have finished discography off – finally.'[37]

'The trouble is, it's convincing for the patient,' says retired spinal surgeon Leigh Atkinson. They can feel the pain, and that convinces them the disc is the source of their trouble. But it's just as possible the pain was caused randomly. The story is the same for other tests that promise to diagnose the cause of back pain, like epidurals or lateral facet blocks. The idea behind those procedures is if you deliver painkiller to a nerve or disc, and that stops the back pain, then you've found the source. 'The surgeon says that's convincing,' says Dr Atkinson. But they don't work either. 'There are a lot of diagnostic tests that are overrated.'

Hence this take from the *Lancet*, one of the world's most respected medical journals: 'No investigation has accurately identified a disc problem as contributing to an individual's pain.'[38] The *Lancet* notes the same problem applies to the facet joints, often identified as a cause of pain: large studies don't show a link between facet joint arthritis and back pain, and we don't have an accurate way of working out if a person's back pain is caused by the facet joints.

Many spine surgeons obviously don't agree with this claim, as it strikes at the heart of their ability to do their job: if you can't reliably identify a painful part of the spine then you can't operate.

As Ashish Diwan, director of the spine service at St George Hospital in Sydney, told me, when it comes to operating on discs to treat back pain, surgeons are working in a large grey area. Once the obvious causes – like instability or deformity, arthritis or compression of the nerves, or narrowing of the channel the spinal cord and nerves run through – are dismissed, the diagnosis of the area that is causing back pain is made based not on absolute data but on pulling together a disparate series of facts. One of those facts, typically, is a patient pushing their surgeon to operate, Dr Diwan says.

'You make a decision based on bits of information, none of which is precise or concise,' he says. 'But … the other alternative is ongoing pain, disability, depression and even offing themselves. The patient tells you they've done everything, spent six months, went to osteopath, chiro. Nothing works, please operate on me. And that is the sort of decision you have to make every day, ten times a day.'

Diwan takes the view that we know the disc can be painful, so we should invest research effort into better tools to find it and treat it. He is working with Dr Kyle Sheldrick to develop an MRI scanning technique that can more accurately pick up disc degeneration, while at the same time working towards a clinical trial of an anti-inflammatory single-molecule treatment targeted directly at the disc.

'Just because we're unable to identify the painful disc doesn't mean the disc is not causing pain,' he tells me.

If successful, the two innovations may radically change the way we treat back pain. But we're not there yet. We have to work with the tools available to us right now. And if you put all the evidence together, the conclusion I come to is: the disc can contribute to back pain. But we don't have a reliable way of picking it out, and, as we'll see, for many cases of back pain that might be being caused by the disc we don't have any reliable treatments.

'The disc can generate pain. It is likely contributing to pain in individuals,' says Jan Hartvigsen, professor of musculoskeletal research at the University of Southern Denmark and lead author of that *Lancet* study. 'What we cannot say, however, is whether it is the cause of pain in an individual patient. Therefore, diagnoses such as "discogenic pain" are meaningless.'

This is the crucial point to keep in mind when you are worrying your back pain is caused by a dodgy disc. It is *possible* bad discs can cause back pain. But we don't have any way of picking a disc causing back pain from one that isn't – or, in fact, differentiating a painful disc from a perfectly healthy one in the spine of a perfectly healthy person.

Ultimately, does it matter? University of New South Wales spine surgeon and researcher Professor Ian Harris does not think so. 'It's mechanistic thinking – that all pain is due to a single, identifiable anatomical lesion. And as soon as we remove it, the pain will immediately cease and never come back again.'

That's too simplistic. Pain is far, far more complex than that.

4   Too much medicine

In 1988, a pair of researchers arrived at a small First Nations community in the Pitjantjatjara homelands.[1] Pitjantjatjara Country stretches across much of the Central Australian Desert, including Uluṟu. The Aṉangu, the researchers wrote, were living quite different lives to the office-working populations of Australia's big cities. Their backs encountered different stresses. The researchers were here, deep in the desert, seeking an answer to an important question. Do non-westernised communities get back pain?

Years later, I asked Peter Honeyman if he remembered his old study. 'I didn't think anyone had ever read it,' he laughs. But then one of his colleagues told him he had read it. 'And it's changed my life,' he told Honeyman.

Indeed, Honeyman's old study has become an important clue to understanding one of the causes of our modern back pain epidemic.

Honeyman tells me the story. Honeyman and his research partner Eva Jacobs interviewed nearly every single person in the community. Most told the researchers they weren't in any pain, including back pain. But, as Jacobs gently built friendships and prodded deeper, many Aṉangu confessed. Actually, their backs did hurt. After putting their data together, the researchers discovered the Aṉangu had back pain – possibly at a rate twice that of Australians living in the big city. But none of these people presented to the clinic with back pain. In only one case did back pain seem to interfere with their lives.

'If doctors ... did not engage in detailed inquiry, they would not discover much back pain in this community. Aboriginal people do not regard back pain as a health issue,' the researchers wrote. A community who experienced a lot of back pain, but did not think of themselves as in pain, and who did not suffer from it. 'None of it seemed to make any sense,' Honeyman now tells me. To Ivan Lin, Honeyman's old study felt like a clue. A hint something else was going on in back pain, beyond the pain bit. A loose thread to tug on.

Dr Lin, a researcher at the University of Western Australia, lives in Geraldton, a small coastal town about 420 kilometres north of Perth. It's a beautiful place, built right up to the water, and when the coastal breezes blow through the streets you could be in paradise. When they don't, it gets so hot it's almost unbearable.

Lin had read Honeyman and Jacob's study. It did not make sense. In between his work at Curtin, Lin works as a physiotherapist for the local Aboriginal health service. His patients were not immune from back pain. Far from it, he tells me. It was ruining their lives. 'I was seeing people who were really disabled, unable to work, unable to take part with their families, avoided doing a heap of stuff they wanted to do,' he says.

Lin led a team of researchers out to three towns in remote Western Australia, deep in the desert, to talk to the local Aboriginal communities about their back pain. A quarter of a century earlier Honeyman and Jacobs found a community just accepted back pain as a temporary part of life, no more serious than a common cold. The attitudes of the 32 people with back pain Lin's team spoke to couldn't have been more different.[2] Over half believed their back pain was caused by damage or wear and tear, most to their spine or the discs. 'They gave me an X-ray of the lower back, and um … it's all worn down,' one man told the team. 'At first I felt a bit weird with them telling me I had arthritis and that. I thought it was a bit of a joke. Then they showed me the X-rays and that and MRI, Cat scan, whatever it was, it was a bit depressing and a bit shocking being young and finding out you've got arthritis,' said another.

How could this be? Perhaps Lin had simply found a group of people with more back pain – entirely possible. Honeyman, remember, was looking at only a single community. But there's another tantalising explanation: perhaps something has changed over the last 30 years about the way these communities saw back pain. Is it possible that what was once an everyday fact of life had been transformed into a disease? 'If what you are told makes you overly fearful of pain, you're likely to rest your back, avoid certain activities – moving, bending, doing the gardening,' says Lin. 'And by avoiding activities, your back becomes deconditioned. And you might become hypervigilant about pain in the back. And that can lead to this spiral of disability.'

Professor Rachelle Buchbinder, a world-leading expert on back pain and overmedicalisation at Monash University, likens it to if we started freaking out about the common cold. 'We know everyone gets back pain – 85 to 90 per cent of us. It's normal. What's not normal is the overmedicalisation. We've really contributed to the burden,' she tells me. The problem is that society and doctors have come to see back pain as a medical problem that needs a medical cure, when nearly always it is not. 'You can see a rise in burden in back pain in Indigenous cultures when they get exposed to western medicine. It suddenly becomes a big medical problem.'

So back pain gets worse when we think of it as a problem and start to try to treat it? Yes, she says. If we turn a normal part of life into a medical diagnosis we strip away our natural resilience, our ability to hang tough when things get tough.

And once you've got a medical problem, I think, people can start making money. Many modern approaches to back pain treatments, both mental and physical, emphasise us taking our healthcare into our own hands. But who profits from that? It's in no one's interest for us to take our problems into our own hands – except us.[3]

The people Lin spoke to hadn't decided their backs were ruined on their own. That view was coming from doctors and chiros and physios, the people they trusted to take care of them. 'The physio and chiro were both saying that it could be a hint of arthritis so I went and got X-rays and I think it was a CAT scan or MRI I had done on my back and then they found out that it was arthritis in the L4, L5 vertebrae. And it hasn't been getting any better since,' a 26-year-old man with disabling chronic lower back pain told the researchers.

A woman told the team her pain was being caused by a slipped disc, with the pain worsening if she moved wrong or lifted something awkwardly. How did she know she had a slipped disc? A doctor told her more than 30 years ago. When you get told your spine is screwed, it tends to stick in your mind. Six of the people Lin's team spoke to said they really feared they were going to end up in a wheelchair. One was just 26 years old – the prime of his life. 'It's the doc that said that, you know if I don't slow down or quit playing sports or whatever, I could, you know, do more damage or end up in a wheelchair or whatever … if I don't have sports I don't really have anything. I feel bored, I don't have life,' said one.

The operations were already starting to mount. One man was preparing for spinal fusion. Another man had had four operations on his back; eventually, his doctor told him it was 'just stuffed'.[4]

Put Honeyman's study together with Lin's, and here's the picture I see emerging: at least some Aboriginal Australians in remote areas once thought of back pain as part of everyday life. As they came more and more into contact with western medicine – with doctors telling them their backs were stuffed – it transformed how they thought about back pain. This explains why the grandchildren of migrants to America are far more likely to have chronic back pain than their parents.[5] When Germany reunified in 1990, West Germany had much higher rates of back pain; over the next 13 years, this gap closed – as back pain levels *increased* in East Germany.[6] And among the people Lin studied, those with the most negative beliefs about their backs also had the highest levels of disability.

This theory explains why people in wealthier countries have much higher rates of back pain than those in developing nations – a situation opposite to many diseases that tend to attack the poorest, and despite the fact more people in low-income nations work in jobs that involve hard physical labour.[7] 'Even Aboriginal people living in remote situations in Australia are not immune to the disabling effects of healthcare,' says Lin. 'And that's the sad thing.'

The typical story of chronic back pain

About six months into researching this book, I began to get confident enough to start bringing it up with people. 'Did you know back pain is one of the largest causes of disability in the world,' I started asking my bemused friends. 'And we don't really know why? And it's maybe got something to do with your brain?'

'Wow,' said Jess. 'You should interview me!'

Jess is the wife of my best friend, Angus. He and I have known each other since first year uni in Adelaide. He met Jess in the alcoholic haze of college induction, and they became close friends and, eventually, partners. After university, I went to Melbourne to take up a cadetship at *The Age*, and Jess and Angus headed for Sydney, where Jess took up a job in architecture. And, occasionally, when Angus called me to catch up and I asked after Jess, he'd mention her back. She's having a bit of trouble right now, he'd say. She's seeing a physio.

So I had some idea Jess had back pain. When I shyly brought up this book, as we sat in a quiet pub in Melbourne, her eyes went wide. Jess, it turned out, was on her own back pain journey. And she was just as lost and scared as anyone else who takes it. This mystery pain had invaded her days and nights, and no one seemed to know how to fix it. She was keen to tell me her story. So we arranged to catch up over the phone, a few weeks later when she was back in Sydney.

'I didn't take it seriously, at first,' she tells me. 'But eventually, it reached a point where I couldn't focus at work. I saw myself unable to travel long distance on planes – and at my worst point, I was starting to see a world where I couldn't work full time. So then I started to take it seriously.'

Jess thinks she first seriously injured her back about five years ago while working in the garden, bending her back to tug weeds from the soil. It was right at the start of her masters in architecture – an extremely stressful and difficult program. Angus remembers barely seeing her that year. The next day her back was so sore she couldn't get out of bed. Before then, she'd had a few minor incidents, stress, soreness, but nothing like this, she said. 'From that point onwards, the back pain has become permanent. And it's grown.'

She managed it for years with regular visits to the physio when things got bad. But two years ago, while slogging through the process of drawing plans for a new building, she developed sharp pains in her arms, neck and upper back. She was later told it was RSI. From there, things became really bad. Her lower and upper back hurt constantly. She struggled to sit or stand comfortably. Her employer paid for an expensive sit–stand desk, but it didn't seem to help. She was missing more and more work. At home, she was struggling with doing housework, while also battling through her final exams to become a registered architect.

She turned to her GP ('who was quite brisk and didn't have much time for me'), who in turn sent her to an exercise physiologist, who prescribed Pilates, which just seemed to make her back sorer. 'I don't think she was very helpful, and

I don't think she took me seriously. She decided I needed to do a lot more exercise – but I'm pretty fit. And the amount of exercise she wanted me to do a day was unrealistic: Pilates, running, on top of what I already do. There's no way you can do that while working full time and maintain a happy life as well.'

Eventually she was referred to a psychologist, who gave her some exercises to deal with stress at work. But she didn't have a cure. No one seemed to be able to tell Jess why her upper and lower back hurt all the time, hurt so bad she couldn't work. 'It's beyond frustrating,' she said. No one seemed to be able to find anything wrong with her. 'So I shouldn't feel this pain. But I do.'

I listened quietly, told her she was brave to speak to me and that her story was pretty heartbreaking. I promised I'd get in touch if I found anything that might help her. But in my head, I was scared. Jess was a smart, healthy, young person, seemingly afflicted by a disease so bad she couldn't work or travel, one that came out of nowhere and took over her life. Doctors couldn't tell her what was wrong. Imagine being like that, I thought to myself. You'd feel like you were stuck down the bottom of a long, dark well, and you'd call for help and no one could help you. You'd feel trapped.

Jess's story has the shape of many others that I've heard from people with chronic back pain. The arc goes like this: a minor, seemingly inconsequential event seems to spark a pain in the back. At first, they think nothing of it. But over weeks and months the pain gets worse. Eventually, they see a GP, who sends them to another specialist, who in turn sends them to another specialist. They try every treatment they can find, each offering little to no relief (and in some cases making them worse). Either no one can tell them what's wrong, or everyone tells them different things. They take time off work, but eventually run short on sick leave or the patience of their boss. Their lives start to fall apart.

Plotted out like that, it looks like a dark spiral, which takes you down and down until you end up asking for – demanding – the last line of treatment: surgery.

The search for a medical cure

This does not fit with how modern medicine is supposed to work. Medicine is filled with miracles. We have drugs that disappear pain and cure disease. We can glue wounds together. We can turn the body's immune system to fight cancer. We can find the problem and apply the solution. Why doesn't back pain work that way?

'The fundamental problem with back pain is there is not a clear connection between damage in the tissues and the experience of pain,' says Professor Paul Hodges, director of the Centre for Clinical Research Excellence in Spinal Pain, Injury and Health at the University of Queensland.

After decades of medical research, we still don't know why 85 to 90 per cent of people get back pain. 'No one knows. Absolutely no one knows. And the people who pretend they know, they are the ones who invent treatments that are counterproductive and create the problem,' says Professor Chris Maher.

For chronic low back pain, in general there is no single highly effective treatment, like a pill that we could take that could cure us. 'As surgeons, we wish we were better at treating it,' says Associate Professor Sarah Olsen.

Yet we still look for a medical cure, flocking to whoever promises one. Indeed, the enormous variety of people offering that cure – chiros and physios, acupuncturists and surgeons – tells us that no one really has something that works 100 per cent of the time.

'If you have any condition that is difficult to pigeonhole, difficult to work out from a diagnostic and even more from a treatment perspective, there's a diverse growth of treatment practitioners,' says neurosurgeon Dr Ralph Mobbs, editor-in-chief of the *Journal of Spine Surgery*. 'And the spine is the best example of that. We don't have a well-established algorithm for how to treat back pain, and we don't have firm treatment algorithms for how we manage it. And therefore there's been this massive growth in the number of people who manage it.'

There's another big problem here, says Mobbs. We know most back pain gets better on its own. That allows all manner of 'snake-oil salesmen' to sell you a treatment – chiro, acupuncture – knowing you'll get better. And when you do, you'll think it was their magic cure, and they'll have locked in a repeat customer. Cha-ching!

We also assume that if medicine can't fix back pain, we should double the dose. We've become obsessed with 'doing something'. This often drives people further down the dark spiral, chasing more and more magical treatments. All these things create a grey zone, where money makers and quacks and people with good intentions but bad evidence come together to make the patient worse, not better.

'If we took away all the harmful treatment, minimised imaging and surgery when it's not appropriate, injecting people, giving them crazy messages, we could *halve* the burden of back pain overnight,' says Professor Mark Hancock.

'Perhaps the biggest problem back pain faces is many of the treatments are *crap,*' says Chris Maher. 'The clearest examples are surgery and opioids.'

We're in a truly bizarre situation, I've come to believe in writing this book. We're gripped by a back pain pandemic – yet many of the world's top back pain researchers are focused not on how to stop the disability caused by back pain, but how to stop their colleagues causing it.

The trouble with scans

Perhaps the best example of why back pain treatments don't follow normal rules is found right at the beginning of the dark spiral, in what might seem like the most unlikely of villains: scans.

When my back pain was at its worst, I asked my physio for an X-ray. I knew something had to be wrong. I wanted to know what it was. I was far from alone. More than 244 000 scans of the lower spine were ordered in Australia in 2021–22, many of them by GPs, who refer more than a quarter of their back pain patients for a scan.[8]

'We feel like if we can see pictures of what's going on, we can fix it,' one GP tells me. 'People like to feel like they've been fully "investigated".'

Getting an X-ray to find out why you've got back pain makes intuitive sense. If a car's engine won't start, we pop the hood. I do this, even though I know absolutely nothing about cars, and have no chance of identifying any likely problem short of the engine being on fire.

Scans can pick out serious problems like spinal tumours, cancer or fractures. But these are extremely rare. If you live in Australia, your chance of turning up to a GP with back pain and it turning out to be something truly awful is very low. One Australian study looked at 1172 people presenting to medicos with low back pain. Just 11 had serious problems.[9] And other than in those rare cases, it cannot help you identify the cause of your back pain.

'An X-ray is useful in so few people,' says Paul Hodges. 'It provides diagnosis in almost nobody. Yet it's given almost routinely. It's a tragedy.' That's why clinical guidelines around the world agree: in general you do not need a scan for lower back pain. Scans can pick up a lot. But they can't pick up *pain*.

OK, fine, you might be thinking. But what's the harm? Even if you don't know anything about cars, popping the hood isn't going to break it. But here's the thing, the weirdness of back pain: scans *can* make you worse. Wrap your head around the results of this randomised controlled trial, published in the *BMJ* in 2001.[10] A team of researchers reached out to 52 GP clinics across England, asking them to enrol anyone who showed up with back pain in a clinical trial. They ended up with 421 people. Half got X-rays. The other half did not. There were no other differences in treatment. That was the whole study. Would it surprise you to learn the people who got X-rays were 26 per cent *more* likely to still have back pain three months later? And they were more disabled? It surprises me.

You can see the same thing in studies on MRIs – more disability in people who pop the hood. And dramatically more spent on future treatments – one study estimated the cost in extra treatments of having an MRI was about US$13 000.[11] Simply getting an MRI makes a person about 30 times more likely to get a course of spinal injections and between 28 and 33 times more likely to get surgery. An MRI sets you up for 'overprescribing, overtesting, intensive and ineffective treatment, and ultimately, poor outcomes', the researchers concluded.[12]

Yet we've become entirely obsessed with them. In one study, soldiers who had back pain were randomised to receive an X-ray. To the scientists' surprise, many soldiers who were told they weren't getting an X-ray snuck off the army base and got one from a doctor anyway.

How can a simple scan make you *worse*? Is the radiation from the scan eating away at our spine? No. The problem with scans is they often start you down back pain's dark spiral.

As we've seen, nearly everyone ends up with some aging and degeneration in their spine. But these changes are normal and natural and largely harmless. 'You see all these disc bulges and prolapses and scary stuff. And you think that's the cause,' James McAuley tells me. 'Everyone has disc bulges. Even things like disc prolapse – people without back pain have some evidence of that.'

The spine's construction does not help. Because X-rays light up bone, not flesh, the spine's vertebrae tend to look like a loosely stacked collection of Jenga blocks, ready to topple at the lightest touch. The X-ray totally misses the huge powerful musculature that holds it all together.

And in the simple act of getting an X-ray and looking at the image, you go from being a person with a sore back to someone who's a patient, part of the medical system. *Medicalised*. You are now sick, rather than strong. 'Imaging will often show up lots of little findings – which are often normal, and aren't linked to the pain. Degenerative changes, for example,' says Dr Hazel Jenkins, who's spent years researching the problems linked to back pain imaging at Macquarie University. 'You can look at a group of patients and they might all have changes – but their pain would be totally different, ranging from no pain to very high pain.'

Is the problem accuracy? I ask Dr Jenkins. 'Not necessarily,' she says. MRIs provide exquisite images of our anatomy. The image is not the problem – it's that most of what we can see simply does not have anything to do with our pain. There is a poor relationship between our anatomy and our back pain.

'If it's used inappropriately, it might send you down this path you did not need to go on,' Dr Jenkins says. 'And if it was managed conservatively, the back pain would have got better on its own.'

Indeed, the negative effects of imaging on back pain seem to get even *worse* with better imaging. Jeffrey Jarvik randomised 380 people with back pain to get either an MRI or an X-ray. A year later, the people who got the MRI were *more* disabled and had had more spinal operations.[13] The same thing can be seen if you look at where MRI machines are distributed across a country – like moths to a flame, the spinal fusions seem to follow.[14]

A huge study of 405 965 Americans who turned up at their GP with back pain, published in 2020, found patients who got an early MRI scan were more than *16 times* more likely to have back surgery and 7 per cent more likely to use opioids.[15] And a year later, the people who had an MRI were in *more pain.*

It gets worse. MRIs are cutting-edge technology, but they are interpreted by humans. And some humans are bad at their jobs. As an experiment, Richard Herzog sent a 63-year-old woman with back and leg pain to have an MRI at ten different practices in New York. They came back with 49 different findings. Not one of them overlapped, across all ten scans.[16]

Unlike popping the hood of a car, having a scan is not entirely without risk – these are, after all, medical procedures. Take the story of Peta Hickey, a 43-year-old senior executive with no history of heart problems. After a work colleague had a heart attack, the office paid for all workers to have CT heart tests. The person who had the initial heart attack recovered, but Hickey had a huge anaphylactic reaction to the CT dye, and died eight days later from multiple organ failure. All from a test she did not need.

In 2014 Chris Maher pulled together the results from the best studies using MRIs to diagnose back pain that he could find. His conclusion: there was no strong evidence the technology could either diagnose someone with back pain or predict someone was going to have back pain.

Despite all this, we spend an extraordinary amount of money on imaging for back pain: about $465 million in 2019–20, according to data from the Australian Institute of Health and Welfare.

'We have this mechanical view of our bodies,' says Professor Flavia Cicuttini, head of the musculoskeletal unit at Monash University. If something hurts, we assume it's broken. We assume we can find the problem on a scan. And then we assume we can fix it with a pill or surgery. But our bodies are not cars or computers. They are living organisms.

They do not abide by the same mechanical rules. 'It reflects our expectations: in 2020, if you're sore, you should have a tablet that fixes it. And these are just normal parts of life,' says Cicuttini.

To get a spinal image is to open a Pandora's box. There really is no way for you or your doctor to know what will leap out from the page and worm its way inside your brain. The discs can look worn, narrowed or blackened. There can be bone-spurs growing off them. It's hard for anyone to look at that and not be a bit worried. It's natural. 'There is always,' writes surgeon Ian Harris in *Surgery, the Ultimate Placebo*, 'something on the MRI report.'[17]

5 'Good posture' – and other back myths

I hold the BackFun in my hands, unsure of quite what I'm supposed to do with it. It's a plastic curve, domed on the bottom, covered in sharp ridges of plastic. It looks like a seat cushion from the Death Star. Mike Phan (not his real name) places the BackFun on the table, where it wobbles and then slowly begins to spin on its hard concave underside. It's black. It's made of what appears to be bullet-resistant kevlar. It looks sort of like a pair of Crocs ... for your butt.

'It's for sitting on,' says Phan, full of enthusiasm. 'Ah,' I say, nodding as though that explains things. 'You sit on it.'

With an enthusiastic wave of his hand, Phan indicates I should stand up and place the BackFun on my seat. I place the BackFun on top of the cafe chair I'm sitting on, steady its slow rotation with my hand, and then gingerly lower myself into it. I feel ... cupped. The BackFun holds my glutes in its half-dome shape. A little spur at the rear encourages a curve in my lower back. Huh. 'It corrects your posture as soon as you sit on it. It corrects your lumbar spine into a natural position,' says Phan.

Phan looks at me expectantly. Unsure of what else to do, I give a little wobble on the dome. Phan grins. The entrepreneur is one of many hoping to make a buck off people with back pain. But Phan's not selling drugs, therapy or surgery. He's selling products to fix your posture. 'There are a lot of studies that have been done on it,' he says. 'Better posture brings better mood, and there's a lot of science behind that. In terms of circulation, in terms of health. Posture, it's where all human balance and life really begins, because it's the connection between your brain and your body.'

The posture market is big business. It started with ergonomics, a field of serious science that has become captured by the manufacturers of varieties of bizarre-looking chairs and unusable-looking computer mice. And now the burgeoning tech field wants to get involved. Phan got his start with the BackFun, which was a hit – he moved four million Death-Star-seat-cushions worldwide. But that's old news. Phan has something new to show me.

It's a shirt that connects to a sensor. The sensor tracks your posture using an accelerometer. The shirt is cut so the material pulls your shoulder blades back and down. The sensor buzzes when it decides your posture is poor. The sensor connects to an app which spits out data on how 'good' your posture was. 'And we'll gamify it!' says Phan. Do well enough and you'll earn 'posture points' which can be used to purchase other posture products, Phan says.

That's not all. You know how wireless headphones often fall out of your ears when you're walking around, asks Phan. I nod, helpless by this stage. Well, the device's sensor will have little hooks that catch them if they fall. Apple have agreed to sell it in their stores.

Posture points. Headphone hooks. It's easy to see why Phan is able to attract funding for his ideas. He's a consummate salesman. I hold up his brochure, thinking. Behind Phan, a large man is leaning over his morning coffee, reading the newspaper. At another table a woman leans back so her waist is almost straight, flicking through the phone in her lap.

'Look at all these people,' I say to Phan. 'They're all sitting differently. And most of these people surely don't have back pain …' 'Most of them do, or will do,' Phan interjects. Well, OK. But how do we know what perfect posture looks like? How does the device decide?

Phan nods sagely, like he's been expecting that one. 'Over 30 per cent of people that go under the knife for back surgery have what we believe to be the myth of the perfect S,' he says, waving his hand to indicate a gently curving spine. 'But for that particular person … that's not that individual's perfect posture.'

It turns out, at least according to Phan, that everyone has a natural inbuilt perfect posture. His device won't have any internal coding for the best posture. You set it yourself. I want to stand like *this* and tilt my shoulders like *this,* you tell the machine, and it'll help you get there. 'Those that suffer from back pain, we live sedentary lifestyles, we sit a lot, we have devices that get you into this hunched position. You're in this locked box inside your body,' says Phan. 'But it's known when you have better posture, when you provide that relief from your back, from the sedentary lifestyles and the tech we're being invaded with, it helps you become better. Posture affects everything. Everything you do.'

This is something we hear all the time. Sit up straight, don't slouch, otherwise you'll end up with a sore back.

But is it true?

'Nah,' posture researcher Chris Swain later tells me. 'That's a load of shit. Sorry.'

There are a few reasons we get back pain. The back is complex, it bears a lot of load, so the muscles can get sore. We bend it into lots of strange shapes every day as we sit and stand, lift and push, run and cycle. To protect it, we're always being told we should worry about our posture. Adjust your computer monitor and desk so everything is at a 90-degree angle! Sit up straight, don't slump! Lift with your knees! Strengthen your core!

Except ... based on the best science we have, none of that is really true. We have woven an incredibly dense web of myth around the back. Some maverick scientists, like James McAuley, have even come to suspect this extraordinary mythmaking – the huge gulf between common sense and evidence – may actually be partially responsible for modern society's back pain epidemic.

We've become a society of hunch-backed mobile phone users. Everyone, every day, spends what must be hours staring at a tiny rectangle, hunched over to read texts or tweets or Facebook messages. It can't be good for us, is the popular wisdom.

But it still came as a shock to many when, in 2019, Australian researchers doing X-ray studies of young mobile phone users discovered in several heavy texters something entirely novel: a pair of tiny bony horns growing upwards and back from the top vertebra in the neck.

'Horns are growing on young people's skulls,' the *Washington Post* headlined. 'Phone use is to blame, research suggests.'

Phone horns! Just the latest risk to young people caused by newfangled technology. 'Now that we see them … growing massively it's quite surprising, particularly finding them in the young generation, when large bone spurs don't normally form before the age of 40 according to the literature,' Dr David Shahar, a University of the Sunshine Coast musculoskeletal researcher, told Nine News. 'The bump is a sign of sustained terrible posture.'

Luckily for us, this is all complete nonsense. Bad science – and really terrible journalism.

The scare was based on a study published in *Scientific Reports* in 2018. The study itself has several problems. First, it lacked a control group of people who didn't use mobile phones, so it's not possible to prove phone use *caused* the bone spurs. Second, the people in the study had visited a clinic *because* of neck pain, so they don't really represent the population as a whole. Oh, and the crucial link between neck horns and phone use – data showing that as you use a phone *more* you are *more likely* to grow horns? Totally unmeasured by the study; it's just a theory put forward by the authors.

Oh, and David Shahar sells posture-related devices at drposture.com, including a pillow that claims to treat forward head posture, a pretty major conflict of interest he failed to declare. (That conflict of interest was later added to the paper.)

Several news outlets immediately debunked the story – but that didn't stop it going viral, notes science journalist Jackson Ryan on *CNet*. It had everything it needed to get going on the internet: a scary headline, panic-mongering about new technologies, and fears about bad posture.

That last bit is key. Throughout history, humans have been obsessed with finding a link between posture and health. One paper I read on posture described it as a 'cultural obsession'. A strong, upright spine has been used by artists and playwrights to suggest strength of character. A hunchback's curved spine communicates weakness or depravity, even evil, medical historian Fay Alberti told the ABC. Leviticus, the third book of the Old Testament, explicitly bans hunchbacks from 'present[ing] food offerings to the Lord'. No surprise then that people with back pain tend to be particularly obsessed with the shape of their spines and jamming them into a 'good posture' compared to those without. They fret about sitting; they fear standing for too long.

Yet here's the thing, the big secret: despite decades of study, *scientists are yet to conclusively prove that posture has anything at all to do with back pain*, nor that there is one particular ideal posture we should be striving for.

'Stand up straight'

On the first day of classes at physiotherapy school, all students are made to strip down to their underwear. It's not a hazing ritual, but it is an initiation of sorts. Unclothed, the students are told to study each other. Look at how each stands. Who slouches? Who has a flat back? Who suffers from forward head position?

Posture, students are taught, is the key to good health and a strong back. It will be their job, when they graduate, to correct it. People with back pain, they are told, tend to have weak muscles in their backs, leaving their spines vulnerable. Get the postural muscles strong and you could cure the back pain.

Some 23 years ago, a young Peter O'Sullivan was standing in that line. He remembers copping it from his instructor: he slouched horribly. 'Stand up straight, man.' O'Sullivan was the wrong person to target. He remembers standing there, shivering, as his classmates ate up their teacher's wisdom about bad posture, thinking: *Says who?*

O'Sullivan's career would be devoted to answering that question. Who says there's such a thing as bad posture? Where's the evidence? He pestered his lecturers. He hunted through research papers. 'And I couldn't find anything,' he tells me. But the accepted wisdom was what it was, and a young physio wasn't in a position to change the world – yet. Anyway, first he had to fix his own back.

As he started his physio course, O'Sullivan had just had a major accident – he'd come off his skis, hard. At first he thought he'd broken his spine. He hadn't, but even after he recovered, the accident left him with chronic back pain. It made standing arduous and bending often impossible. Even as he worked his way through university and started out as a practising physio, O'Sullivan was thinking he wouldn't be able to last in the job.

Eventually, at his lowest point, O'Sullivan spied himself by chance in the mirror. There he was, standing as straight as he could, core on, guarding his back against further injury. He looked, he thought to himself, completely ridiculous. If he was going to have back pain, he wasn't going to have it looking stupid and feeling stressed – especially because, he remembered, there really wasn't any evidence it was important.

O'Sullivan quit holding himself so upright. He allowed his natural slouch to creep back in. He *relaxed*. And, little by little, the pain went away.

That's an anecdote, O'Sullivan tells me, laughing. You can't make science out of anecdote. But O'Sullivan was hooked. He knew the evidence for posture was crap – and he'd just cured himself by quitting trying to stand up straight. He decided to re-enrol at university and research posture.

First, O'Sullivan led a team of researchers who conducted a proper, formal search for evidence that posture made a difference to back pain or general health. They found none. Then they started doing their own studies. First they studied people's postures when they sat, looking at whether they slumped or not. They found no association between sitting posture and back pain. 'There's this kind of fear. My god, if you slouch, you're going to end up with pain, you'll end up hunched over. We just don't have evidence to support that.'

'There is just no good evidence' that posture is in any way a problem, O'Sullivan says. 'Often, this is a distractor from the big game. Our spinal health is linked to our general health. Keeping fit and strong. Moving. Eating well. Sleeping well. They're the things we should be targeting. Rather than this idea of targeting body posture. The interventions that have targeted posture haven't worked. We have to look beyond that.'

O'Sullivan's ideas troubled me at first because they are so *radical*. How could posture not matter? But he enjoys widespread support from leaders in pain science. 'He's a very much respected person in the pain space. He's done an enormous amount of work,' says Tim Austin, chair of the Australian Physiotherapy Association's National Pain Group. 'Peter is on the mark.'

Your posture is governed by the slow-twitch muscle fibres that run through your back. They're designed to hold positions for a long period of time, but eventually become fatigued. Under stress, they tend to get short and tight. People who don't move around much tend to overuse these muscles and underuse their more athletic fast-twitch muscles.

What posture should we hold them in? Straight, you might think. But this seems an odd idea, given the spine is naturally curved like an S. Mechanically, it's just not designed to be straight, says sports and exercise physiotherapist Andrew Smythe. If all the vertebrae were stacked neatly atop one another, there would be tremendous pressure in the bottom components. The S shape is like a suspension bridge, holding thousands of cars aloft by a gossamer thread: it evenly distributes the load across the spine.

'But the precise S-curve of your spine is individual to you. It's in your genes,' says O'Sullivan. 'Look around a room. Look at the variability of how people hold themselves. It's like our signature. It's just how we are. This idea of homogenising us, I think it's more social.'

So where does it come from? Historian Sander Gilman thinks it comes out of the military: the military pose of 'standing at attention', spine rigid, chin tucked, feet under head.[1] This was originally developed as the ideal pose for reloading a musket, and was never natural. Soldiers have to practise it again and again to master it. Over time, this posture became imbued with manliness and honour, and non-soldiers started trying to imitate it. Now we're all trying to stand to attention – despite there being no scientific evidence it's good for us.

In a study of 1108 Australian teenagers using photographic analysis of sitting posture, researchers could find no association between posture and the incidence of headache or neck pain.[2] In adults, there is some evidence of an association between forward head position and neck pain – but it's not clear which way causation runs.[3] Do we maintain a forward head position because we're in pain, or does the position cause the pain?

What about back pain? Again, despite dozens of studies, no strong evidence has emerged for a link between posture and back pain, according to an umbrella review of the evidence.[4] Even in people who are forced to take on awkward postures for work, there is no evidence this increases the risk of back pain.[5]

Part of the issue is scientific. 'It's really difficult to measure the different types of physical loads that are placed on the spine. Even changing your posture a little bit can change how the loads are distributed quite a lot,' says Chris Swain, the researcher who led the metanalysis.

So we can't *precisely* measure the effect of posture on back pain. But, says Swain, there are now enough studies coming to similar conclusions that we can come to an *imprecise* conclusion: posture likely doesn't matter, and if it does matter, the effect is very small.

'The association just isn't that strong,' says Swain. Compare it to things that really make a difference, like depression and anxiety, and the evidence suggests posture just isn't worth worrying about for most people, he says. 'I'm fairly slouched now – and I don't worry about it.'

There is some evidence people with chronic back pain have weak back muscles. When you image them, you can see the muscle has become withered and infiltrated by strands of white fat. It's not clear yet why this is. But it doesn't seem crucial to back pain, because when doctors devised special training programs to strengthen those muscles they found they didn't help anyone's back pain.

'At an undergrad physio level, they talk about ideal posture and biomechanics,' physiotherapist Andrew Smythe tells me. Then, after really getting to grips with the research, 'you kind of see it's all bullshit'. If you're healthy, posture just does not seem to matter that much. 'It's the same with running. Look at some of the best runners in the world – they have really funky techniques that don't fit the textbook, but structurally and functionally they're strong,' says Smythe.

Smythe tells me he gets parents bringing their children in to see him over concerns about their posture. Yet the bemused kids aren't in any pain. That's just their natural posture. Smythe checks them over for any red flags before turning his attention to the real problem: the panicked parent.

Brendan Mouatt is director of a physiotherapy and exercise physiology practice in Melbourne called The Biomechanics. When he was starting out, biomechanics seemed the solution to all back pain problems. 'Get their posture right and they won't have any pain,' he tells me. 'But what we see now is none of those factors have to change for people to improve. There was a big focus on biomechanical research for a while – and now there's starting to be a big shift away.' The name is going to have to change, he tells me with a sigh.

Of course, there's no evidence sitting up straight is actually *bad* for you, experts said. If you feel comfortable that way, or think you look better, go for it. The problems can arise when people are *worried* about their posture. 'It's probably more the anxiety, the fear of not being able to get in that [straight] position, thinking there's something wrong with them,' says Smythe. 'They can spiral into "I should have pain because I don't have a good back" – and that's sometimes where those horrible chronic pain cases can start.'

There's one area where posture does seem to make a difference: movement. But it's not the posture we hold, it's the movement between postures. In several studies, researchers have found a link between people who don't move much between different sitting postures over the course of a day and back pain. The idea seems to be that there is no one ideal posture, but that our bodies do best when they're regularly moving between different postures, straining and working different muscles.

Indeed, this is probably why we get sore if we sit the same way for too long: not because we're damaging our backs, but because our pain system is telling us to *move, please*. Why? Our cells are constantly taking in nutrients from our blood and pushing out waste products, some of which can be quite acidic. It could be that sitting in one pose too long allows all those nasties to build up; moving, which increases our heart rate, literally flushes out our system.

After panicked headlines (inaccurately) proclaiming sitting was the 'new smoking', modern offices have embraced sit–stand desks. But Smythe and his colleagues aren't seeing any fewer injuries. Standing in a static position places as much stress on the body as sitting in one. Once again, movement is key.

'Strengthen your core'

Posture is one back pain obsession. The second is the core – the slabs of muscle that corset our torso and support and stabilise the spine and pelvis; think abs, but also the lower back and the muscles that wrap around our hips. They play a role in basically everything we do, every twist and bend and lift and lunge, we are repeatedly told. They allow power to transfer from lower to upper body. A strong core is a ticket to six-pack abs and a bullet-proof back. Even the name sounds seductive. An apple without a core is just a husk. The core provides foundation for everything else we do in life.

'Your core muscles are the base of support for your entire body,' personal trainer Meredith McHale told *Shape* magazine in 2018. 'A strong core helps keep a more upright and erect posture whether you're being active or just sitting at your desk.'[6] Strength coach Kristina Jennings told the same article that a 'weak core is the number-one risk for potential injuries, especially lower-back injuries.' The number one cause! The theory runs that a strong core cradles the spine in a way that protects it from injury; a weak core, or one that has not been trained to turn on at the right times, leaves the spine vulnerable.

An obsession with the core has always been deeply coded into western society. Catherine de Medici, queen of France in the 16th century, is credited with making the corset popular in Europe, where iron and whalebone reduced a woman's waist to just 50 centimetres, and led to an outbreak of women fainting at balls.[7] Men were for a long time allowed to wear their fat with pride, but in the early 19th century that too shifted as a new obsession with the muscled marbles of ancient Greece led to strong, muscular bodies becoming desired. The birth of bodybuilding in the 20th century eventually led us to today, where movies tell men that having a six-pack is normal and expected. 'You'll ask people, what do you reckon is the cause of the pain: "Oh, my posture is crap and I've got a weak core",' says O'Sullivan. 'Almost everybody tells me that.'

This was the social background. Then in 2004 a scientific paper came along and lit the fuse.

The researchers used electrodes on the surface of the skin and implanted into the muscle to measure how the core muscles fired as volunteers moved their arms. In the people with low back pain, the researchers found, the transverse abdominus – the deepest layer of abdominal muscle – fired notably later than in healthy controls. Their cores were weak, and that was contributing to instability and back pain, the study seemed to suggest.[8]

The paper was 'huge', says O'Sullivan. People already believed a strong core was important to health – and now they had a paper to prove it. The findings reverberated through the physiotherapy profession and out into gyms and glossy magazines around the world.

The problem was the study did not hold up to scrutiny. It was tiny: just 14 people with back pain were tested. 'They identified milliseconds in timing difference in a muscle

– and they were extrapolating that to say this muscle is deficient. It was a small signal, but the extrapolation just kind of flooded the market,' says O'Sullivan. And the research was extremely difficult to do. The researchers had to push fine wire electrodes a couple of centimetres into the volunteers' chests; when O'Sullivan tried to replicate the experiment one of his subjects fainted in pain – they ended up having to abandon the project.

In 2010, Swiss researchers finally managed to recreate the original experiment. But, in a much larger trial, they couldn't find any link between core activation and back pain.[9] But that paper was too little, too late. The genie was already out of the bottle. The original paper has now been cited almost 1000 times; the Swiss trial, just 44.

While all this was happening, Paul Marshall was working through an exercise physiology PhD at Western Sydney University. Obviously he was going to study the core. Marshall wanted to build the perfect core exercise program. A series of moves that worked the hip, trunk and abdomen, activating all the right muscles, laying a flawless foundation of strength. Marshall was confident the program would work. He'd spoken to all the experts, read all the latest research. 'We thought it was perfect,' Marshall says. 'We were chasing the magical exercise.'

The results of the clinical trial were heartbreaking. Marshall's perfect core exercise program did no better in cutting back pain than just asking people to get moving. All that work, it seemed, for naught.

Marshall went back to the drawing board. Was the program wrong? Were there exercises he'd missed? After much puzzling, Marshall was forced to come to a new conclusion: training the core simply didn't seem to matter. *Exercise* was what mattered. 'The core aspects of motor control, they'll change regardless of the type of exercise you do. It doesn't need to be all this core abdominal work,' he told me. 'It's a consistent theme in the literature. These problems, when we talk about the abdominal muscles – they seem to change regardless of what we do.'

Up in Perth, Peter O'Sullivan had caught the core stability bug too. He wanted to find a core muscle program that would treat back pain. 'We were trying to train them to activate these muscles. Some were saying, when they were doing this, that it was making their pain worse. They couldn't breathe, it was just making them feel stiff. And I remember just looking at them – they were looking robotic in the way they were moving, and I was thinking, *This can't be right.* It's not normal to be walking around sucking your tummy in all the time. It's not normal to be constantly contracting muscles.'

Having these muscles turned on all the time seemed to act as a signal, or a reminder, to the people to constantly think about the back, and back pain – and we now know, says O'Sullivan, that pain hypervigilance is only going to make the pain worse. Indeed, when O'Sullivan looked at his results, he found many of the people with chronic back pain had *overactive* core musculature. O'Sullivan was trying to get them to turn on their cores, but they were already in overdrive. 'They were already overworking these muscles. Typically we see people over-guard the core when they're in pain.'

In another study, O'Sullivan showed the average healthy person did not turn on their core at all when they lifted things. They just … lifted. No switching on the abs, nothing. The only people turning on their core were the people in pain. 'We were training people to do something that wasn't normal,' O'Sullivan says.

Many people do find training their core muscles helps their back pain. We shouldn't dismiss that. But a lot of that may be down to building confidence in their body, or just moving more in general. Multiple meta-analyses fail to find a significant benefit for core stability training over a standard exercise program in the long term.[10] We're actually getting to the point now where scientists are starting to conclude we don't need to do any more research: it simply works no better than any other exercise program. 'The trials that have trained patients with back pain to work their core, any benefits from those … are more related to having more confidence in your body. It's not related to the thing you're doing,' says O'Sullivan.

Again, much as with posture, O'Sullivan isn't saying core stability exercising is bad. It does help some people; others tend to get better anyway. But overall, the evidence simply does not support worrying about it too much, he says. 'Planks, push-ups, sit-ups. That's fine for the back. But this idea of bracing the core when you move, that's not normal.'

'Lift with your knees'

Alf Nachemson is a huge figure in back pain – one of the most influential spine scientists of the 20th century.[11] He helped transform the science of back pain from a mechanical one to one that understood the pain was often a symptom of a much more complex issue involving psychology, sociology and the brain.[12] He also did a lot of work to push back pain into the modern era of evidence-based medicine, and was one of the founders of the vitally important Cochrane back review group.

But one of Nachemson's greatest legacies – he died in 2006 at the age of 75 – may prove wrong.[13] You see, Nachemson is at least partially responsible for the way we lift things. That classic stance – quite awkward if you think about it – with back straight, legs bent, bum out, pushing the weight through our legs and butt.

His studies in the 1950s and '60s popularised the idea that a straight back was important while lifting, and that otherwise the back was at risk of injury. Just about every work health and safety course in the country teaches the method. It may seem to be common sense.

But it might not be true.

Alf Nachemson was never trying to find the safest way to lift something. He wanted to understand the basic bio-mechanics of the spine – something scientists did not really have a firm grasp on in the '60s, when he was working. At the time, everyone agreed the disc was the cause of back pain, but no one had been able to prove exactly how it caused agony.[14]

In his lab at the University of Uppsala, he rigged a thin metal catheter to an pressure gauge – a bit like the needle on a bike pump. Somehow, Nachemson managed to secure a supply of fresh spines, taken out of people who had died in the last few days. The surgeon sliced away the muscle and bone, cutting the spine down to only a single disc. Then Nachemson placed the disc in a vice and inserted his pressure needle.

As Nachemson increased pressure to the vice and started squeezing the disc, the needle wobbled and ticked upward as pressure inside the disc increased. Enough pressure and the disc dissolved into a bloody pulp. The fairly predictable result of crushing something in a vice, you might say.

Nachemson then moved onto actual, living people. His catheter almost immediately broke off in the spine of one of his first volunteers. Expecting to get sued, Nachemson went home and told his wife to pack her bags for Sweden.

But Nachemson did not get sued. Instead, the study turned him into one of back pain's most important – and most misinterpreted – figures.

Nachemson eventually got his technique right and started measuring the pressure in living, moving humans.[15] His first experiment was on posture. 'Bend forward, please,' he told his volunteers, while watching the needle on his pressure gauge rise and rise. More measurements were made with the subjects holding weights.

These experiments and more like them eventually allowed Nachemson to draw up a little chart of pressure on the disc in different postures. Its most famous depiction – you might have seen it on the wall of a doctor – is of a little series of pressure graphs, with a tiny, sad-looking figure depicted atop each one in the corresponding pose.

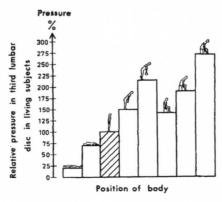

It's pretty easy for you and me to interpret these studies. The spine is strongest when it is straight. For each degree of bend, the pressure on each disc dramatically increases. These results and this neat little diagram have been overinterpreted by generations of doctors and physios, who point to it to warn their patients about the dangers of bending over too far.

'Basically, Nachemson described how when you're in a bent position the pressure in the disc goes up,' says O'Sullivan, who has studied the history of the straight-back myth. 'Others translated his work to "If there's more pressure in the structure, it must make it more vulnerable to injury". This long bow was extrapolated from this data.

'It's almost like Chinese whispers – one gets fed on another, and then it becomes the truth. As a physio student, I was educated on this. And once something becomes the truth, it's so hard to pedal back from. So anyone who might question it is seen to be ridiculous.'

Nachemson measured the disc pressure caused by different postures. But his study does not show that different loads, or different postures, cause damage or pain to the disc. It might make sense that adding load to a disc would increase the chances of damaging it, but – as we see again and again with back pain – just because something seems to make sense does not mean it is true.

In late 2019, a team of researchers in Australia published a review looking at all the evidence for the safety of lifting with a straight back instead of a rounded back.[16] Their findings: there was none. 'There is no evidence that lifting with a flexed or round back increases your risk of back pain,' says O'Sullivan – who, as you're coming to appreciate, loves to make trouble.

'In fact, people with back pain were more likely keep their back *straighter* when they lifted,' adds Nic Saraceni, his PhD student, who co-authored the review.

The study, published in the *Journal of Orthopaedic and Sports Physical Therapy*, pulled together data from 12 studies, totalling almost 697 people. After pooling the results, the team could not find evidence suggesting one type of lift put you at greater risk for back pain. There is *not enough evidence* to say lifting with a straight back is best – which is strange, given how widespread the advice is.

'It seems like such a well-known thing – everyone knows to lift with a straight back. You'd think there'd be really strong evidence to support it,' says Saraceni. 'But there's just not that much data.'

The results might surprise you, but they did not surprise David Hall, a workplace safety specialist and the spokesperson for the Australian Physiotherapy Association. 'We've known this for decades,' he told me. 'The emphasis on keeping the back straight is a bit of a dogma that's lasted through the ages. It's like the idea you should sit bolt upright at a computer – that's not true either.'

Some 50 years later, we have no evidence lifting with a rounded back, or a slumped posture, puts the back at risk. Near the end of his life, in 2006, Nachemson told an interviewer from *Spine* those earlier studies had been misinterpreted.

'This experiment has been misinterpreted as evidence that the disc is a significant pain generator and that increasing the biomechanical load leads to greater pain,' Nachemson told *Spine*. 'But this study merely showed how the lumbar spine responds to normal physiologic loading in various positions of the body. It does not give any indication as to where the pain actually comes from.'[17]

Far from advocating for a spine held firm and straight, Nachemson's later work led him to become a huge advocate of spinal motion – which he believed promoted better blood flow and nutrition to the discs. To protect his spine, he even became an avid jogger.

There's no scientific basis for ergonomics

Posture. The core. Lifting with a straight back. These are three pillars of our back myths. The fourth encompasses all three – and, once the veil of myth is lifted, is perhaps the most maddening: ergonomics.

Ergonomics is the scientific discipline responsible for some of the more bizarre fads we see sweep in and out of offices. Strangely shaped chairs and angular computer mice. And now, everywhere, the sit–stand desk. My newspaper must have spent a mint replacing the entire staff's desks with sit–stands, most of which – after a single joyride up and down – now remain static in exactly the same posture as the old, non-mobile desks. The company and most others employ people, or contract them in, to perform 'ergonomic assessments', moving the chair height and keyboard layout just so, so our elbows and knees make neat right angles.

It's big business. It's hard to get firm figures on how big the industry is, but the Australian office supply market is tipped to generate \$10.1 billion in revenue this year, according to IBISWorld. The firm's analysts believe the slice of that supplied by the ergonomics industry is rapidly increasing. That fits with three ergonomics firms I spoke to, who all said the industry had enjoyed explosive growth in the last 15 years.

But here's the thing: there is simply no evidence ergonomics is anything more than nonsense. 'Ergonomics does not have a firm basis in science', says Professor Chris Maher.

He has been telling ergonomists for years that most of their interventions lack evidence to show they work. They don't want to hear it, he says: 'I've been astonished that the ergonomics industry has been allowed to get away with this for so long.' Ergonomics is a science, meaning it's supposed to be based on evidence. But many standard 'ergonomic interventions', like the desk adjustments that nearly every office worker has experienced, lack evidence to show that they work.

'I think it's a load of rubbish,' says Associate Professor James McAuley. Peter O'Sullivan laughs when asked about ergonomics's scientific support: 'This thing, it's built like a house of cards.'

Perhaps the strongest evidence against ergonomics comes from our friends at Cochrane. Five times they've looked directly at ergonomics: for carpal tunnel syndrome and for preventing and treating work-related arm, neck and shoulder pain. Using an 'alternative' mouse combined with a shoulder support probably reduced the risk of neck and shoulder disorders, although alternative mice did nothing on their own. Beyond that, they could not find strong evidence showing *any* of the interventions worked.

A 2015 review published in the leading *British Medical Journal* managed to discover some moderate strength evidence that having someone adjust your desk or monitor *did not work at all*. These 'adjustments' are the 'bread and butter' of what ergonomists are called in for, one leading consultancy told me.

Maher is blunt: 'It's an area of research that's littered with bad studies. And once you ignore the bad studies, you're left with studies showing it does not work.'

Standing desks: 'There's no evidence they're effective for controlling work-related musculoskeletal disorders.'

Ergonomic redesigns of the workplace: 'We don't know if that works.'

Interventions to cut back pain: 'People still think about fancy chairs, fancy desks. If you're going to invest in trying to cut back pain, your best bet is to do … exercises. That's the only thing that's got evidence for it.'

About 15 years ago, an unusual invitation dropped on Maher's desk. The nation's ergonomists were having a conference in Cairns, and they wondered if he would speak.

Maher took the room through the evidence. There was, he said, almost none. 'I did not get very well received,' he says drily. 'People didn't talk to me at morning tea. But my job is to summarise the evidence that's out there. I don't have vested interests in this area. I'm paid by the government as a researcher.' Maher has spent close to two decades building a database of high-quality empirical research for a range of physiotherapy treatments. He is yet to see a rigorous study that supports ergonomics.

O'Sullivan calls ergonomics 'the science of belief. You can have pain associated with sitting, but it doesn't mean the way you sit caused it', he says. 'The evidence, as I've seen it, suggests ergonomic interventions are no more effective than non-ergonomic interventions. They haven't reduced the burden of back and neck pain.'

But ergonomics is more than just dodgy science. Its core ideas – that a bad mouse, or the wrong chair, or a poorly adjusted desk can injure you – have seeped into mainstream social consciousness. What do they tell us? That our bodies and, in particular, backs are weak and easily injured by simply sitting wrong.

'It promotes the idea there's a correct way to sit. That's just rubbish. There's no correct way to sit,' says McAuley. 'In our research we see people all the time who've been advised to sit up straight at their desk. This has just made their pain worse. As far as preventing musculoskeletal pain goes, I think that ergonomics is rubbish. I think it's possibly dangerous.'

Confronted with all this evidence, Australia's ergonomics society admitted to me that yes, they have some big problems. 'If someone attempts to deal with back pain for a sedentary worker, and all they do is adjust their seat height and add a bit of lumbar support, not only have they missed the point, but they clearly don't understand the fine points of applied low back biomechanics and they obviously have no idea what practising effective ergonomics is all about,' says Stephen Hehir, chair of the Human Factors and Ergonomics Society of Australia's professional affairs board.

A desk adjustment wasn't ergonomics at all, he added, and the 'right-angle erect seated posture promoted by some in the furniture industry' was simply wrong. But he said the analyses that suggested a lack of evidence for ergonomic interventions were flawed. Many of the studies, like Cochrane's, weren't published in leading ergonomics journals, and most of the interventions they tested weren't done by qualified ergonomists, he said. 'Imagine if they were reviewing surgical outcomes and including [people] operating without a medical licence rather than only qualified surgeons,' he said.

Despite the lack of evidence for ergonomics being an actual science, ergonomists are still regularly called on as expert witnesses. I found a number of cases in court records where ergonomists testify on whether workplace design, furniture or practice might have contributed to an injury. One ergonomics consultancy told me they saw 'hundreds and hundreds' of cases a year. 'We're asked for ergonomic opinions as to what happened and why and what could have been done to prevent it. When they show they weren't shown how to do things properly, they win more than they lose,' the veteran consultant said.

Maher says, 'I'd be concerned if the ergonomist gave advice that a poor office or desk set-up caused or contributed to a worker's injury because we just don't have the evidence to support such a statement.'

Lisa-Maree Cakir is one worker who was awarded tribunal-ordered compensation – after she suffered an injury *caused by* an ergonomics intervention. Cakir was working as a web publishing officer with the Department of Employment and Workplace Relations when she was given an 'ergonomic assessment of [her] workstation' by an injury management consultant, according to tribunal papers.

The consultant performed a desk adjustment on her workstation, and then prescribed her an S-Board, one of the dozens of different types of ergonomic keyboard. They're much smaller than a normal keyboard, allowing the mouse to sit closer to the keys, which is supposed to be good for the shoulders. Cakir told her supervisor it made her neck and shoulders ache. Her department's health and safety officer told her to keep using it for a few more weeks, tribunal papers show. But her pain grew and grew, until she had to go on extended sick leave.

She later asked Comcare, the public service workers' compensation insurer, for compensation for the injury, then took them to the Administrative Appeals Tribunal when they rejected her claim.

She alleged the S-Board and a 'poor ergonomic set-up' led to her injury. Comcare argued the 'workstation was ergonomically assessed by a suitably qualified person and ergonomically approved equipment was provided, and it is simply implausible to claim that an injury resulted from these changes'. The tribunal disagreed, finding her injuries came from the S-Board and 'changes in the ergonomic arrangement of her workstation', and ordered Comcare to compensate her and pay her costs.

Ergonomists who spoke to me almost universally acknowledged the field has an evidence problem. They have different suggestions as to why. 'One of the reasons there's not gold standard evidence for ergonomics is because it's unethical not to do ergonomics,' says ergonomist Leon Straker. Because the field believes ergonomics works, deliberately putting someone in an un-ergonomic environment would be unethical. Hence, it is argued, you cannot test if it truly works.

And pain from working at a desk is a lot harder to measure than, say, whether you have cancer or not. Capturing improvements in tiny signals is another real challenge for ergonomic studies, says Straker.

Critics aren't buying it.

'It's nonsense. There are trials with interventions that are way more complex than this,' says Maher. 'We do placebo-controlled trials of surgery. Those people who say it can't be done, they're ignoring the studies that have been done but come back negative.'

In an effort to close this gap, University of Queensland Associate Professor Venerina Johnston and her colleagues set out to conduct a proper randomised trial on ergonomic interventions to reduce the impact of neck pain in office workers. They split a pool of 763 office workers into two groups. The first group received an ergonomic adjustment of their desk plus some health education, while the second got the adjustment and a program of neck exercises. Remarkably, workers in both groups took more sick leave after the intervention started than they had before, and productivity loss increased.

'Generally, ergonomic interventions don't show much change in terms of musculoskeletal problems,' Johnston concludes.

Alf Nachemson, who we met earlier, was hailed as the 'godfather' of ergonomics by the journal *Spine* – remember his work showing some sitting postures were less harmful to the spine than others? By the end of his career, he'd become one of the field's fiercest critics. Nachemson told his interviewer that, based on early ergonomics studies, he and his team had redesigned an entire car manufacturing plant for Volvo to minimise stress on the spine. It didn't work – at all. Puzzled, Nachemson did a later study at the aircraft manufacturer Boeing, looking at what physical factors at work might cause back pain. The strongest predictor? Psychological risk factors, not physical ones.

'This study opened my eyes, and those of the world, to the fact that back pain isn't only about the spine, it is also about the brain,' Nachemson told *Spine*.

How we think about backs

All of this nonsense – posture, core strength, ergonomics – leads us to perhaps the most radical idea I've come across in back pain, one that really got me interested in writing this book. Bad posture and a weak core and a badly set-up desk don't really seem to put you at risk of back pain. But the way we *think about them* just might.

In the last decade, radical ideas about back pain's causes have started to gain momentum. A group of scientists believe that our back pain epidemic is being caused not by something physically wrong with our spines but by something *culturally wrong with our beliefs*: how we think about our backs and how we think about back pain. A cultural illness. A society-wide sickness of how we think and speak.

Like a plague, it's transmitted mouth to mouth, but also by our media and sometimes by the very people we look to to take care of us. An idea that's a virus. If we could take that virus and put its DNA under the microscope, here's what the base pairs would spell out:

Spines are fragile. Backs are weak. Lift something wrong and you can hurt them. The pain you feel is a sign something has gone physically wrong. And when damage is done, it only gets worse over time. Stand wrong and you can hurt your back. Sit wrong and you can hurt your back. Wear the wrong damn schoolbag and you can injure yourself.

These myths have become deeply embedded in our culture. In one study done in New Zealand in 2014, almost 90 per cent of people said it was 'easy to injure your back'.[18] Some 98 per cent of people agreed that good posture was important to protect your back. Almost 90 per cent believed it was important not to ignore back pain because that could cause long-term damage to the back.

'What do we think about backs in our western culture? We think they often get fragile as you get a bit older. And [that] they're not very strong, really. And [that] it's something that really should be protected,' says James McAuley. 'And the more you worry about that stuff, the more likely you are to get back pain.'

The link between pain and belief

Early research on pain and belief emerged from studies on hypnosis – which, far from being a sideshow carnival attraction, is actually highly studied for its ability to alter a person's beliefs about themselves.

Hypnosis has a long history in treating and preventing pain; way back in the 1840s hypnotists reported using hypnosis to anaesthetise patients during surgeries.[19] Modern science shows it really works. One brain imaging study showed that a hypnotist's suggestion of pain in the hand led to both a feeling of pain *and* activity in several regions of the brain associated with feeling pain.

In several randomised controlled trials, hypnosis has shown improvements over usual care for chronic pain management. Hypnosis has even been shown to be somewhat effective in reducing pain in people with sore backs.[20]

If we can edit a person's beliefs and affect their pain experience, well, what are all the messages about our backs being fragile doing to us?

'Human beliefs are so hard to overcome. We're belief-driven. We're fundamentally not evidence-driven creatures,' says Peter O'Sullivan.

It's not much of a leap to suggest that an idea could slide into the brain and prime it. And then, when we inevitably do have back pain, the scene is set for the brain to become very, very worried about what's going on.

Perversely, worrying about posture and core strength might actually make us more likely to have back pain, several scientists argue. Anxiety is strongly linked to back pain. And society primes us with message after message about the importance of posture to protect your back – like Mike Phan's BackFun.

'The messaging around pain, that it might be related to your posture – well, people will get anxious. And it will make pain worse,' says Chris Swain, the posture researcher.

Can *beliefs* about backs really make us more likely to hurt them? One obvious problematic belief is that our spines are fragile. If we worry our spines are fragile, we're going to move them less. With less movement, the muscles that hold our spines aloft atrophy – perversely putting them more at risk of injury.

'Belief is really important. It's so tightly interlinked with our behaviour,' says exercise physiologist Brendan Mouatt. 'I see lots of people who believe "I've got my mother's knees", or "I think this is genetic – my parents have always had this". … There's a component there that influences how we view our spines, what they're supposed to do.'

There's evidence to show this is exactly what's happening. In 2008 Associate Professor Donna Urquhart and a team from Monash University recruited 192 ordinary people and surveyed them about how they thought about back pain.[21] Is back pain permanent, they asked? If you have a bad back once, will you always have a bad back? Can a bad back eventually put you in a wheelchair?

The researchers followed the volunteers over two years, looking at who went on to develop back pain. The people who started out with more negative beliefs at the start of the study, the team found, were more likely to experience serious back pain over the next two years.

All the negative cultural and personal beliefs about our backs feed into what pain scientist Professor Lorimer Moseley believes is a vicious cycle. 'If you're convinced pain equals damage, you get more pain, so you think you're getting more damage, so your brain gives you more pain, so you think you're getting even more damage,' he says. He thinks the trigger for most back pain is an injury, although often only a small one. But because our culture has fetishised the weakness of the back, in some people that's enough to send them into a spin.

'People don't just twist their back,' he says. 'People twist their ankles. But when it's your back, you *wrack* it. Exactly the same injury. And from then on it's a "dodgy back".' People believe a fractured arm will miraculously heal, but a sprained back won't. 'Tissues heal. It's an irresistible, unstoppable force of biology,' says Moseley. (We'll hear a lot more from Lorimer Moseley in a later chapter.)

So every time we feel a jolt of pain in our backs, it signals to our brain – primed with all the worst-case-scenario messages about back pain – that the damage is getting worse. The brain, anxious and confused, ramps up the pain, sending panicked signals that *something is bad and something needs to be done about it.* As the pain gets worse, you think your spine is falling apart.

We digest and incorporate these ideas about pain early. You can see this learning process going on in the face of every child who has fallen over and skinned a knee. The child's brain is trying to work out how threatening the injury is, and it does this by looking at Mum or Dad. Ever noticed how a child might fall over but won't cry until a parent comes rushing in to hug them better? That's the *signal* that they're hurting, they're injured, they're unsafe.

'We grow up with this idea that "If my knee bleeds a little bit, I'll have a bit of pain. And if the tissue has been damaged more, I'll have more pain",' says Joshua Pate, a pain scientist based at the University of Technology Sydney. 'We grow up thinking pain is in proportion to damage. Pain is about protection. It's about how much threat is needing to be addressed, rather than how broken am I.'

Pate has done a lot of working interviewing kids about how they think about pain. He sees the same thing again and again. One kid, asked about knee pain, said matter-of-factly that the right treatment for knee pain was a knee replacement. It turned out his mum had just had one. 'That's the kind of scaffolding that happens throughout childhood,' says Pate.

Indeed, our society as a whole doesn't handle pain very well. We avoid it at all costs. We hide from it with drugs. We *fear* it. That may be why we're so bad at handling what is a normal part of life. 'We're scared of pain. No one wants to feel it. But it's a part of life. Whether it's emotional or physical, it's there. Having that is how we appreciate the contrast of feeling happy, appreciating life. You can't have one without the other,' says pain psychologist Jess Chu. 'We can't avoid it. Unless you're born with a deficit in your brain in that area, you're going to feel pain.'

If all these beliefs really matter to back pain, we should be able to prove it. Because we humans are remarkably gullible and our beliefs are fairly easy to manipulate; the entire behemoth advertising industry is built on that insight. We should be able to design an experiment to change people's beliefs about back pain and then see if it changes how much pain they suffer.

Archived and nearly forgotten, just such an experiment exists.

In 1997 WorkCover, Victoria's workers' safety regulator, launched 'Back Pain – Don't Take It Lying Down', a multi-million-dollar experiment in the power of belief. WorkCover got interested because, then as now, back pain makes up an enormous amount of workers' injury claims; nearly 50 per cent of all claim payouts were for back pain in 1997. Those costs had tripled over the last decade, and the agency was at a loss as to how to stop them.

Watching the ads now, they're of their time – grainy, the men in ill-fitting suits – but the messages still resonate. 'The human spine is surprisingly difficult to damage,' says a spine surgeon. 'It's very unlikely you'll ever need spinal surgery.' The surgeon's message is powerful and important.

It's an ad that even I can remember from watching TV as a nine year old.

It stars Merv Hughes, one of Australia's most iconic cricketers, a wonderful fast bowler, heavy drinker, and owner of a giant horseshoe moustache. Hughes was also well known, like many fast bowlers, as a sufferer of back pain. The ad starts with Hughes in full cricket gear, wearing a wide-brimmed hat while fielding close to the boundary. He stretches his back side to side and, tickled, the entire crowd behind him mimics the strange movement. 'People used to think I was fooling around out there with those exercises,' Hughes says. 'What they didn't realise was, I've got a disc bulge that gives me a lot of pain. And it would give me a lot more pain if I didn't give it a lot of exercise. So, if you've got back pain, give exercise a go,' says Hughes, and then flings down a ball, slicing through a hapless batsman's wicket.

The ads ran during prime time, often during breaks from the football or cricket, along with radio and print ads, billboards, posters and workplace visits. The core messages were simple: stay active, keep going to work, don't lie in bed. 'That was about really trying to get at the fundamental misconceptions people have: that physical activity will make it worse, that you should rest, that it would inevitably get worse, that you won't be able to work. We know being active and working is actually better for you,' Rachelle Buchbinder, who was deeply involved in the ads' formulation, tells me. 'We primed people. So when they got an episode of back pain, they knew it was going to get better.'

Surveys run after the campaign suggested it was working. Nearly everyone could remember the ad, and 89 per cent understood the core message: if your back hurts, keep moving and stay active. To measure how well the ad campaign worked, Buchbinder's team measured the beliefs around back pain in Victoria and then compared them to people in New South Wales, where the ad did not air. Their study showed big changes in Victorians' belief about back pain, and no changes in New South Wales at all. Perhaps more importantly, Buchbinder found her ads changed how *doctors* and back pain specialists thought about and treated back pain.

And what about the result? Did claims for back pain drop? Yes – and dramatically. Compensation claims for back pain dropped 15 per cent, time off work fell, and WorkCover recorded an overall 20 per cent cut in their compensation costs.[20]

'And now for the kicker,' writes Buchbinder in the book she wrote with surgeon Ian Harris, *Hippocrasy.* 'One group of people wasn't affected by the campaign at all.'[23] The doctors who said they *knew the most* about back pain. The specialists. The people who, Buchbinder found, were often giving out the *worst* treatment for back pain, encouraging people to stay in bed, ordering expensive scans. They 'did not shift their beliefs in the slightest', she writes. 'The bottom line? If you have low back pain, avoid seeing doctors who declare a special interest in it.'

The evidence suggests people saw the back pain ads, changed their *beliefs,* and that led to a drop in the number of people struggling with chronic back pain. This is amazing, right? We've now got campaigns like this running all around the world, right?

Buchbinder wanted $300 000 every two years for a maintenance campaign to keep the ideas fresh in people's minds – chump change compared to how much WorkCover had saved. But in 1999, Victoria's state government changed. Jeff Kennett's Liberal party was replaced in a landslide by Steve Bracks's Labor government.

At the same time, says Buchbinder, WorkCover's entire board turned over, many leaving for the Australian Wheat Board (where, in a further twist, they were soon embroiled in an oil-for-wheat scandal after being caught paying kickbacks to Iraqi dictator Saddam Hussein). Despite the positive results, the new board displayed little interest in the ads.

'No one wanted to be associated with the old board, so they stopped the ads. And the government didn't want to be associated with the old government, so they didn't want to do them. It was really stupid,' says Buchbinder. They cheaped out, contracting a media company to run a few ineffectual ads. After that, everyone lost interest. And the idea, like so many good ones, died. The original copies of the ads – which really do seem to have changed how Victorians think about back pain *and* cut how much they were suffering – now likely sit in some dusty archive at WorkCover. 'They don't even know they own the ads. It's a huge missed opportunity,' says Buchbinder.

6 Pain and profit

In 2014, a visitor darkened the doorway of Dr Roy Carey. Carey is a veteran spine surgeon; he's seen more 30 000 private patients over his career and spent a couple of years as president of the Spine Society of Australia. But what distinguishes Carey most, I think, is his willingness to speak the truth – even when it gets him into trouble, and even when it annoys his colleagues.

Carey's visitor was from Bupa, the health insurance giant. Later, a manager at WorkSafe Victoria would also pay the veteran surgeon a visit. They both told Carey the same story: the amount they were paying out for spinal surgery was going up and up and up. The insurers wanted Carey to work out what was going on.

Carey got to work. He assembled a team of seven top spinal surgeons, asked WorkSafe for a random sample of 300 spinal fusion bills, and began to review them.

'And that's when you start to see what other people charge for things,' Dr Carey says to me. 'And I thought "F---. I could have been on my fourth Maserati by now."'

I looked up. Dr Carey was staring at at me wide-eyed over my notepad. 'Inappropriate and fraudulent' practices are now rampant, he says. 'We've allowed Dracula to drink freely from the blood bank.'

Spinal fusion – the biggest money maker

Spine surgery, and in particular spinal fusion, is a lucrative area of medicine on its own. When you add in what Dr Carey would spend the next few years revealing – years of inappropriate billing to Medicare and private health insurers – it becomes extraordinarily lucrative.

The first thing Dr Carey's team noticed: the average number of item numbers – a unique code for each operation, each attracting a different government subsidy – billed per fusion was 11. Some had as many as 19 different item numbers. 'Things that were plainly impossible – like a code for operating from the back of the spine when it was done from the front,' Carey says.

Those codes are sent to Services Australia, which oversees Medicare. The subsidy then gets paid back to the surgeon. No checking. It's a trust-based system, says Carey. 'Bupa said to me "We just didn't think surgeons would do this".'

What about the private health insurers? Surely they would complain. But by law, private health insurers must pay out on items that Medicare pays out on. Medicare pays, and therefore insurers must. 'It's the perfect crime. Patients don't know. Surgeons orchestrate. Private health insurers can't do anything,' Carey says.

And most patients, of course, don't know enough about Medicare item numbers to ever question whether their bill is right. If they've got private health insurance, the bill is often sent straight to the insurer.

Governments that don't ask. Patients that don't know. Surgeons raking in the cash. 'This really is the perfect crime!' I say to Carey. He laughs.

Worse was to come when Dr Carey's team looked at Bupa's receipts. Of the roughly 1200 spinal fusions they reviewed in 2018, more than 85 per cent of the bills had inappropriate claims. Carey is not shy about what this is: 'scamming', he labelled it in a 2020 article in the Australian Orthopaedic Association's newsletter. We will never know just how much money has been fraudulently taken from Medicare over the years, he claims.

But this is only half the story. By carefully reviewing patient case notes, Carey's team also discovered that many of the operations were themselves inappropriate. 'We found, of that 300, we would have approved – give me a guess,' he says.

'Um – two hundred?' I hazard.

'No. Seven.'

'*No.*'

'Two hundred and ninety-three of the first three hundred we considered to be inappropriate.'

WorkSafe were so concerned with Dr Carey's findings that they established their own surgical review board, made up of seven spinal surgeons, to check whether patients being booked in by surgeons for fusion really needed one. Between the middle of 2018 and the end of 2019, the panel supported 328 fusion decisions – and knocked back 316, a knock-back rate of 49 per cent. Extrapolate that to non-WorkSafe surgeons and we have an awful lot of inappropriate fusions being done. 'Medicine,' says Carey as I wrap the interview, 'is now a business, not a profession.'

And business is booming. Across the the world you can see an explosion in the number of expensive things being done to sore backs. America, where profit is king, is by far the worst example.[1] Spinal MRI rates rose 307 per cent between 1994 and 2004. Steroid injections into the back were up 623-odd per cent. Spinal fusion increased by something like 220 per cent. Spine surgery is simply out of control, writes Dr David Hanscom, an American complex spine surgeon for 32 years, in *Do You Really Need Spine Surgery?*[2]

In Australia's healthcare system, surgeons don't face the same extreme pressures to make profit – but the industry still faces similar problems.

'We have an unregulated industry that can do whatever it wants. And we have a fee-for-service model,' says Chris Maher, the University of Sydney's back pain expert.

Spinal fusion rates here jumped 167 per cent in the private hospital sector between 1997 and 2006 – a rate of growth much higher than hip or knee surgery.[3] In the public sector, that growth rate was just 2 per cent. Data that Carey says Bupa provided him with show spinal fusion *costs* rose 36 per cent between 2011–12 and 2014–15.

'The thing I see in it is money – extraordinary amounts of money,' says Lorraine Long, head of Australia's Medical Error Action Group. 'Was the operation necessary? The private hospitals, they don't care. It's money coming in.'

Make no mistake, spinal fusions are extraordinarily expensive procedures – among the biggest money makers in a spinal surgeon's workbook. And the surgeons earn far, far more operating on privately insured patients, which may explain why the surgery is more than ten times more likely to happen in the private rather than the public system.

Plus many surgeons receive large rebates on many of the items used in the surgery, paid by the big medical device companies that sell them, says Dr Rachel David,

CEO of Private Healthcare Australia. She told me she's been approached by several spine surgeons who have complained of their colleagues attempting 'heroic' (read: enormous) fusions over two surgical sessions, which doubles the rebate earned – and keeps the patient in hospital longer, allowing the private hospitals themselves to profit.

Every part of spinal fusions has become a source of profit. The surgical screws themselves cost about US$1000, at least ten times the cost of making them, Reed Hastings reported in the *New York Times*. In some cases, Hastings reported, doctors took ownership stakes in the companies making and selling these screws – and then installed the screws in their patients.

The practice, or something like it, has spread to Australia. One surgeon operating on Australia's east coast offers a financial disclosure form that lists financial relationships, including royalties, with companies selling cages used in spinal fusions and with a physiotherapy practice that the surgeon refers patients to.

Spend half an hour with sources from within the multinational medical device industry, as I did while researching this section, and you look at medicine – and surgery, in particular – in an entirely different light. One salesman I interviewed told me that after one particularly painful round of negotiations with the federal government on behalf of his company he came home and told his wife he felt like he worked for Big Tobacco.

'The prices we pay here are too high,' he tells me. 'And the companies don't pay their fair share of tax.'

Here's how the industry works. Medical device companies spend thousands of dollars to sponsor medical conventions and other industry days, where they set out booths to display their latest wares. This is where they hunt for connections. 'When you're selling to surgeons, you're constantly trying to build a relationship,' says another source. The surgeon agrees to try out some of the company's products in surgery. So the sales representative turns up – often to the surprise of the patient – in surgery. 'As a device sales representative, you're in theatre every single day. Helping with cases, trying to sell them more,' says the same source.

After some time 'assisting in theatre' to build that relationship of trust, the representative might start subtly introducing new products. 'We're getting really good patient outcomes with this new artificial disc – have you seen our new trial?' Another potential sale. This does not cost the patient anything – their private health insurance pays.

My source tells me that the surgeons themselves don't make money off this – they're usually motivated by the thought of helping their patients. The problem is the companies and sales staff don't share those goals. They're often there to make money. 'It's not about patient outcomes if you're not hitting your [sales] numbers,' says another source. There are only so many surgeons to sell to, so companies often aim to increase the *number* of operations done – trying out a course of epidural steroids before a spinal fusion, for example, or adding a bone graft substitute to a spinal fusion operation.

A good spinal surgeon might be worth $1 million-plus in sales and profit to a company, so they get the royal treatment. 'The best way to think of a surgeon is a high roller in a casino,' says one source. A surgeon who uses a lot of a company's products might get flown to expensive international conferences in Paris or Rome, where they give presentations on their surgical technique, which just happens to make heavy use of the company's products. 'What you get is the fame, the ego,' says the source. Have a research project you'd love to undertake? The device company will fund it. Maybe the company is working on a new device – would you like to be a co-designer for a component of the royalties? Some companies even sign up surgeons as paid consultants – and then, suddenly, that surgeon switches all his business to the device company.

You can see then, why Curtin University pain psychologist Dr Rob Schütze tells me that 'chronic back pain feels like a political and a moral problem'. 'You've got people taking advantage,' he continues. 'And maybe not malevolently or in a calculated way, but they do at some level know better. And they're taking advantage of people who are very vulnerable, who are desperate. And we can do better.'

Spine surgeon Ian Harris tells me he doesn't think his colleagues are knowingly doing surgeries that don't work. 'I don't believe a homeopath wakes up in the morning and heads to work thinking he's going to rip off another 20 customers.' The problem is, they often don't understand the evidence – or choose to ignore it. Many surgeons, Harris says, are more interested in the technical aspects of surgery, not the patient outcomes. 'They live in a bubble.'

Regardless of motive, the more we spend the worse we feel. One study in the US state of Maine found the best surgical outcomes occurred when back surgery rates were lowest. The more people treated, the worse the outcomes.

Other treatments that don't work

This is the real tragedy of back pain. The vast majority of treatments lack scientific evidence to show they work reliably. In many cases, we have good evidence they *do not* work. And yet we continue to pay for them.

'The reflex is to do something,' writes Nortin Hadler in *Stabbed in the Back*. 'The more dramatic something is, particularly if it is dangerous and painful, the more it is accepted by peers and held in awe by laity.'[4]

Jabs

Leslie Abboud is a medical negligence lawyer based in Sydney. He's been in the game for 35 years, and sounds exactly how you'd expect a malpractice lawyer to sound: wry, and deeply cynical about the medical profession.

About a third of the 10 000 cases he's taken are related to people injured in spinal operations. A lot of them are people who've been badly injured by an epidural steroid injection to treat chronic low back pain. Painkilling injections, steroids meant to cut inflammation, facet-joint jabs – 'all that shit,' says Abboud. 'It's a good way for the radiologist to make money,' he says. 'They think it doesn't cause much harm. But there's so much risk with those injections.'

Epidural steroid injections involve a steroid shot into the epidural space, the tiny canal the delicate spinal nerves run through.[5] The theory is that the steroid reduces inflammation in the area; local anaesthetic can also be used. They have become enormously popular tools for people suffering back pain, their use more than doubling between 2001 and 2011; about 40 000 Australians a year line up for a shot.[6] Many doctors, under pressure to wean their patients off opioids, have resorted to them.

In her meticulously researched back pain best-seller *Crooked*, American investigative journalist CJ Ramin links the explosion in the use of these injections to entrepreneurial American anaesthetists.[7] When the insurers they were billing discovered most of the procedures they were involved in could be handed off to nurses, the more entrepreneurial and underemployed of their number reinvented themselves as interventional pain physicians, selling a menu of nerve blocks and Botox and steroid jabs, despite 'knowing little about treating musculoskeletal disorders'.

Because they're cheap, easy, attractive and 'low risk', they are being done 'willy-nilly', says Abboud. Take one of Abboud's recent cases: a woman who received 22 jabs in a year to deal with back pain. The Mayo Clinic suggests you should get no more than three or four a year; this woman was turned into a pincushion.

In another case, one of Abboud's clients received an epidural injection to treat lower back pain at a medical imaging clinic in Western Sydney. After the injection, the back pain got much worse, and he felt severe heaviness in his legs. Later that night, at home, the man discovered his legs had become completely paralysed. Doctors soon discovered his spinal cord and spine itself had been damaged because the needle had been inserted into the wrong place. Abboud got him hundreds of thousands in compensation, but he now walks with a limp and lives with constant pain.

Maree Rivero took her GP's advice and consented to a course of epidural steroid injections. Rivero is a research and development manager, and she read through the evidence beforehand. 'It was a bit mixed,' she told me, 'but I put my faith in my GP.' He'd had back pain before, he said, and knew how to treat it.

She now regrets that faith. Her GP decided to perform the injections himself at his small regional hospital. After the injection, the nursing staff took her out to a small waiting room for observation. She lay down to rest. She remembers being tired and sore. She remembers the nursing staff telling her it was time to go home, and sitting her up.

She does not remember the next bit, but found out about it later. The GP's needle had missed the target and sliced through the outer lining on her spinal cord. Cerebrospinal fluid started leaking into the surrounding tissues. With the fluid leaking out, the pressure in her brain cavity was dropping. When she sat up, it fell dramatically. 'It was like being hit over the back of the head with a cricket bat,' says Rivero. She had that same headache for the next month.

How do they fix a leak in your spinal cord? I asked.

You have to have the same procedure all over again. They draw some of your own blood, plunge the needle into the original site of the damage, squirt the blood in and hope it seals up the hole. It doesn't always work. Maree needed two goes. 'I trusted my GP,' says Rivero. 'And I shouldn't have.' He later told her he'd done thousands of injections, and hers was the only spinal cord he'd nicked.

Steroid injections are generally considered safe, but the risk is not zero.[8] Reported side effects from injections include headache, dizziness, pain, and pins and needles. More serious side effects are sometimes caused by the medico misplacing the needle and puncturing something important. These include compression of nerve roots in the spine, infection of the disc, a build-up of pus in the spinal cord, and even paraplegia.

In 2013, Pfizer grew so concerned about the off-label use of one of their anti-inflammatory drugs, Depo-Medrol, as a spinal injection that they asked regulators around the world to ban its use in epidurals, citing a risk of 'blindness, stroke, paralysis and death', according to the *New York Times*. Australia's TGA and regulators around the world did so; America's FDA did not. In a bid to tackle the opioid epidemic, America's politicians even approved a boosted rebate for the procedure, encouraging pain clinics to turn into 'drill mills', in the words of one critic.

But perhaps the most troubling side effect of steroids is on the bones. Glucocorticosteroids are known to mess with the metabolism of your very-much-alive bones, decreasing the rate at which new bone is formed. In a study of 3000 Americans who received a lumbar epidural steroid injection, researchers showed that each injection *increased the risk of bone fracture by around 20 per cent.*

All these risks might be worth it if the injections worked. Multiple reviews of trials, including one from Cochrane, have found they are no better than placebo injections – simple shots of saline.[9] It doesn't seem to matter what type of back pain you have, or where you're injected, they just don't work. A review of 30 trials, published in the *Annals of Internal Medicine* in 2015, found small short-term benefits for low back pain – so small they might not even matter to many people.[10] People often feel better after receiving one, but that's likely to be a placebo effect, or even the back pain just naturally getting better on its own. The story is the same for sciatica: a benefit so marginal you might not even notice.[11]

'These injections are bad science and bad medicine,' spine surgeon Ian Harris told the *Australian Financial Review* in 2014. Guidelines from the Australian and New Zealand Association of Neurologists strongly recommend against using them for back pain when there's no pain radiating down into the legs, because even though the risks are small, they do not outweigh the benefits. Which are zero.

And here's the kicker. Many patients try epidural steroids as a front-line option, thinking they might help (unlikely), don't come with any risks (not quite) and could be a good alternative to surgery. Sadly, the evidence suggests this does not happen: having a course of shots does not make you any less likely to end up under the knife.[12]

That mirrors my father's experience. His second injection provided calming relief (the first did nothing). 'The surgeon said it would be like getting a rest, taking a break,' said Dad, 'and it was. I could breathe. But the pain came back, just like he said it would, and I had surgery.'

Intradiscal electrothermal annuloplasty (IDET)

Intradiscal electrothermal annuloplasty is another in the long line of treatments designed to treat degenerative discs[13] – all which seem to ignore the evidence that (a) people can have blackened, gnarled discs and not be in any pain, and

(b) even if a disc is causing pain, we don't have any good test to work out which one it is.

Anyway. IDET, as it is known, inserts a catheter into a 'painful' disc, and then slowly heats it to 90 degrees Celsius. It will remain this hot for about four minutes. This, we are told, is a 'non-invasive therapy'.

IDET was introduced in the year 2000 by back pain specialists who were inspired by cauterisation, where surgeons burn some tissue to essentially seal a wound.[14] Could the same thing be done to a damaged disc? they wondered. In experiments on animals they showed that heat could shrink the disc, a bit like what happens when you burn cling wrap.

At first, results looked incredibly promising.[15] The first study reported a success rate of around 75 per cent. Even better, the trial reported zero side effects. Zero!

Clinical trial results that are too good to be true should raise big red flags – especially in things as hard to treat as back pain. The studies were essentially reporting that you could use a hot needle to burn someone's disc without anything going wrong – not just that, but that their new trick could cure chronic back pain, something no one else was having much success with. But instead of raising red flags, the paper was accepted for publication in the field's leading journal *Spine*.

Everyone became very excited, especially as other surgeons started replicating the results in their own practices.[16] 'It's like the disc has a facelift. We get rid of the wrinkles and cracks so that it works better,' one London spine surgeon told the *Daily Mail* back in 2001 when the procedure was growing popular.

That first paper does not mention, as far as I can tell, that the inventors stood to gain financially from their device. Other IDET papers obliquely noted 'benefits in some form have been or will be received from a commercial party related directly or indirectly to the subject of this manuscript'.[17]

Nortin Hadler was an editorial board member of *Spine* at the time. 'I had no idea of the extent of the commercial involvement,' he writes. The inventors founded a company. By 2001, it was turning over $21 million annually from IDET products. It was later sold for $310 million.

The inventors were publishing results, incredibly good ones, about a device sold by a company one of them co-founded.[18]

'If this was a pharmaceutical, it would never have been licensed on the basis of such information,' writes Hadler in *Stabbed in the Back*.

Enter Christopher Cain. 'If it sounds too good to be true,' he tells me, 'it usually is.' Cain is now a professor in the spine division of the University of Colorado, Denver, but back in 2005 he was working as a spine surgeon in the department of orthopaedics at the Royal Adelaide Hospital. He and his colleagues did not buy the evidence the inventors were selling. 'They were fairly anecdotal. They weren't good scientific studies,' he says.

This scepticism caused quite a fuss, given IDET was becoming very popular. It was marketed as non-invasive, it seemed safe, and it was relatively cheap, so its use was taking off. 'Medicine is a business,' says Cain. 'It's a business of recruiting patients for treatments to generate revenue for hospitals and doctors. Sometimes it's hard to differentiate the financial benefit to the providers from the benefit to the patient in terms of relieving symptoms.'

The inventors met the scepticism head-on. You don't believe us? they said. OK – let's do a proper study. With funding from their company, Cain and his colleagues put together a very careful experiment. Patients with back pain of exactly the type the inventors said IDET would treat were randomised into two groups. One group received the procedure. The other simply had the catheter inserted but not turned on. Because of the anaesthetic used and the careful set-up in the operating room, neither group was able to tell whether they received the treatment.

When the results came in, the improvement shown in earlier studies disappeared. If there was any improvement, it was so slim as to be attributable to statistical noise – and sometimes patients got worse. The inventors weren't happy. They pushed the surgeons to change the experiment parameters, look at patients with less damage to their discs. 'But even when we looked at those patients, there was still no difference,' says Cain. 'It did not work at all. There is really very little benefit beyond the placebo effect.'

Then there were the side effects. Cain calls it a low-risk procedure, but things do go wrong. Sometimes the catheter got stuck in the disc and broke off – requiring extensive surgery to remove. Sometimes the catheter damaged a nerve. Sometimes the punctured, burnt disc developed an infection. Sometimes you got a cerebral spinal fluid leak. The technique seems to weaken the disc, increasing the chances of a hernia.[19] One study reported complication rates as high as 15 per cent – much higher than the zero reported in the first study.

IDET is meant to shrink the disc like burning cling wrap. But sometimes it blows up the disc to giant proportions. That happened to a 29-year-old soldier, who turned up at a medical centre after spending a year and a half fighting chronic back pain that radiated into his left thigh. He'd tried everything: chiropractors, opioids, injections. The surgeons decided to apply IDET to two discs that were showing small signs of deterioration. The procedure went perfectly, the surgeons reported. But the soldier came back a few days later – the pain was now much worse than before. The surgeons opted to bump up his opioid doses. Several weeks later, he was back again, eventually convincing the doctors to MRI his spine. The disc had responded to IDET by blowing up, a huge mushroom of dead and damaged material pushing into the delicate spinal cord. The patient – now hooked on fentanyl – was booked in for a spinal fusion; the surgeons spent much of the procedure picking apart the ballooned disc.

Perhaps the worst complication I have come across: in rare cases, the heat can get high enough to cause bone surrounding the disc to die, eventually leading to accelerated disc degeneration and bone collapse.

'If a surgeon proposes it – and there are plenty of places that still offer it – you should ask "Would you undergo this procedure yourself?"' says Cain. 'I would not have it done. I would not recommend anyone I care about have it done.'

Radiofrequency denervation

Radiofrequency denervation has a lot of similarities to IDET – although, while IDET has somewhat fallen by the wayside, many enthusiasts of 'nerve burning' remain. A needle is inserted at the supposed site of pain – often the facet joints, sometimes the discs themselves – where it is pushed up against nerves thought to be transmitting the pain. The needle is then heated with a burst of electricity or radiation. The heat kills the nerve and, theoretically, ends the pain.

As far as scientists can tell, it also does not work.

Denervation has an incredible history.[20] It starts in 1914, when a young Vincent Nesfield of the Indian Medical Service was stationed on the front lines of World War I in Mesopotamia. Soldiers kept coming to Nesfield's infirmary with 'trench back', back pain caused after a trench collapsed on them. Nesfield decided the problem was a hooked nerve somehow tangled in a muscle or tendon, and determined to cut it free.

He took a thin, long, curved scalpel and made cuts down both sides of the soldiers' spines, moving the blade back and forth vertically. The treatment was an apparent success, though Nesfield wouldn't get much of a chance to exploit it – he was soon deregistered by medical authorities for trying to hawk a miracle injection he called 'Vitalexin'. But by then he'd already passed on the trick to British surgeon William Skyrme Rees. Rees wouldn't last as a doctor either – he was drummed out after penning an official report claiming British hospitals were the dirtiest in the world. Rees took the trip many ostracised people do: to the Antipodes. He hung out a shingle in the tiny New South Wales town of Tocumwal and started slicing into the spines of farmers with back pain.

Rees penned a letter to an academic journal announcing

that he had cured 998 of the first 1000 patients he'd seen – causing a huge stir nationally and internationally. Better, Rees had come to the attention of the then federal health minister Dr Doug Everingham, who was so enamoured of the doctor's treatment that he installed an extremely high government rebate for the procedure.

Rees, now famous, moved to Macquarie Street, started giving lectures, and became a media darling, now claiming Nesfield's spine-slicing as his own invention. It wasn't until 1977 that other surgeons seriously studied what Rees was doing and discovered that, far from slicing a nerve, the scalpel was slicing into muscle. If the muscle was spasming, the cut likely relieved some of the spasm (Rees completely rejected that claim).

That takes us up to 1972, when Rees had a fortuitous meeting with C Norman Shealy, an American neurosurgeon who was fresh off inventing the implantable spinal cord stimulator. Shealy tested Rees's technique and found it led to too much bleeding for his taste; he replaced the scalpel with electrodes, and radiofrequency denervation was born. Shealy reported a 90 per cent success rate, and back pain doctors once again had a new toy to play with. The procedure took off in popularity and has never stopped.

In a story that will now be familiar to you, it took until 2001 – 25 years after the procedure had been pioneered – for good quality placebo-controlled evidence to be published. Richard Leclaire and his team inserted a catheter into the spine of 70 patients, but only half of the group of 70 patients got a *hot* catheter.[21] The results were straightforward. After four weeks there were no differences in pain, disability, flexibility or strength between the two groups. Whether the nerve was burnt or not seemed to make no difference. A Cochrane review in 2015 concluded there was no high-quality evidence showing the procedure worked at all for chronic low back pain.[22]

The failure of the procedure is borne out in repeat rates; about a third of people who have one ablation will have another within three years, suggesting that if they do provide relief, it is temporary at best.

'How many more waves of therapeutic zeal must we witness – waves of spine-surgical inventiveness that provide nothing more than testimony to hubris and often greed – before we design a way to abort the next?' asks Nortin Hadler in *Stabbed in the Back*.[23]

The problem is how expensive it is to run a proper clinical trial of a new surgical intervention. Why would a company or a treatment pioneer spend millions of dollars to potentially discover their money-making procedure does not work? As patients, this leaves us exposed to medical treatments that are often tested far too late. 'This is a big problem in medicine,' says Dr Ralph Mobbs. 'And I don't know the answer.'

Spine surgeon Ian Harris is far less charitable. 'There's no burden of proof on surgeons,' he tells me. 'In surgery, we think up things to do, and we continue to do them until someone goes out of their way to go and do a study to find out if it works or not. There's no requirement to do the study.'

After writing about all the damage done by inventive procedures given to tens of thousands of people before ever being properly tested, I'm inclined to agree with him.

By now, you may be getting sick of this rogues' gallery of failed treatments and harmed patients. But pay particular attention to this one. I think nerve burning is a clue, a signal among the wreckage of failed back pain treatments that tells us that something *strange* is going on here.

Nerve burning cuts the transmissions between sensory nerve and brain. If that sensory nerve is in a painful area, the pain should stop, right? But it doesn't. The pain keeps on and on, despite the cable being severed.

'It assumes there's a direct, one-to-one relationship between pain and sensory nerve information,' says Dr Matthew Bagg, a back pain researcher at NeuRA (Neuroscience Research Australia) who has studied the therapy. 'And we know that's just not the case.'

7   Big pharma

Emma Phillips has dark red hair, pale skin, a proud chin, dark, focused eyes. She was given the nerve pain drug Lyrica to help with her viral meningitis, a painful inflammation of the spinal cord caused by an infection. Lyrica, the brand name for pregabalin, is not indicated for its management.

Her doctor never took a mental health history. If he had, he would have found out Emma already suffered from depression. Perhaps then he wouldn't have prescribed the drug – or at least, hopefully, he would have warned her that pregabalin's side effects included depression, and suicidal thoughts.

'I had severe changes in mental health. Severe. Severe. You are not the same person,' she told me. 'It's really, really scary. There's a feeling of complete worthlessness. It makes you feel like you don't deserve to be here. I was looking at my veins. I was looking at knives.'

Ms Phillips is one of tens of thousands of Australians put on pregabalin in recent years, as the drug has exploded into one of the country's most popular medicines. Many of those prescriptions appear to have been written for back pain, making the pregabalin crisis a back pain crisis. I spent much of 2017 uncovering the story of Lyrica. The story I eventually wound up with is really a small-scale retelling of the back pain story in general: a dubious treatment pushed by a big pharma company that stands to make hundreds of millions of dollars. Patients encouraged to ask for it, and doctors far too willing to prescribe it. And huge amounts of harm done before anyone looks to make sure the drug is helping, not harming.

The story of Lyrica

Lyrica, sadly, is really just a repeat of the opioid cycle. Indeed, the growth of Lyrica was fuelled in part by doctors seeking a safer alternative to opioids. Pfizer initially said Lyrica was not addictive, a claim that now appears to be false.

In 2011 few had heard of Lyrica. It was mostly confined to specialist pain clinics, doses kept low to minimise nasty side effects. Eight years later, it is one of Australia's most prescribed drugs. More than 4 million scripts for pregabalin were written in 2017–18, up from 36 242 in 2011–12.

'Now everyone is on it for everything,' Professor Rachelle Buchbinder told me. 'I spend my whole day taking people off it.'

How did it become a blockbuster? Via a sophisticated and well-funded effort by Pfizer to win a government subsidy for the drug, then promote it to doctors and consumers. 'It was an absolutely superior marketing effort on Pfizer's part,' says Lesley Brydon of Painaustralia, the peak national body for chronic pain. 'And it was multi-pronged. They looked at their community, and said "How can we play a role here to get this on the PBS?" They did it in a very strategic way, which embraced all the key influencers. It was a sophisticated marketing strategy.'

None of Pfizer's actions are illegal. But the story of Lyrica reveals the enormous influence pharmaceutical companies like Pfizer can have. In 2010, chronic pain wasn't on the agenda in Australia. There were few specialist doctors, no code number for chronic pain in hospitals, and few effective medicines available. Painaustralia was launched to advocate for those affected. Ms Brydon became its founding CEO.

Meanwhile, Pfizer had a drug for treating nerve pain: pregabalin. But it was expensive, and, according to some experts, not much better than a placebo for some common pain conditions like sciatica. In 2011, the health department rejected Pfizer's application for a taxpayer subsidy for Lyrica because of 'uncertain cost effectiveness'.

Health consumer organisations are meant to represent the interests of patients, lobby for funding for conditions, and fight for new drugs to be made available. But many accept significant donations from pharmaceutical companies, putting them at risk of a conflict of interests.

Pfizer gave Painaustralia $433 175 between 2011 and 2016, according to Pfizer's disclosure records. (Painaustralia puts this figure at $247 000.) Two other health consumer groups, Chronic Pain Australia and the Australian Pain Management Association, each got hundreds of thousands of dollars too.

Spokespeople for all three groups denied that Pfizer's funding – which they said was untied and unconditional – influenced them in any way. The funding was used for newsletters, education, media campaigns and other activities, and each said they never lobbied on Pfizer's behalf. But Ms Brydon, who retired from Painaustralia in 2017, was happy to speak candidly. 'It was part of their marketing strategy. They wouldn't have done it otherwise. Why would they do it otherwise?' she asked.

A Pfizer spokesman said all its relationships were firmly above board. 'Health consumer organisations play a vital role in supporting patients, their families and carers living with difficult health conditions, as well as advocating for improved standards of care and access to treatments,' the spokesman said. 'Pfizer's relationships with these groups are based on integrity, respect, and transparency, ensuring the independence and credibility of both organisations. We firmly contest any insinuation to the contrary.'

Pfizer also supported the National Pain Summit at Parliament House in Canberra in 2010, as well as the development of Painaustralia's national pain strategy. That strategy – with a foreword by a scientist who is a speaker for Pfizer and who took part in a Pfizer-funded trial on Lyrica, alongside Pfizer's employees – called for Lyrica and other chronic pain medicines to be subsidised.

In 2012, Pfizer applied for a subsidy again. When a drug company applies for a subsidy, consumer groups are invited to make submissions. These submissions, which are meant to represent the views of patients, can have enormous influence on subsidy decisions, experts told me. The Australian Pain Management Association made a submission to the department, I discovered; Chronic Pain Australia encouraged its members to do the same. As mentioned earlier, both groups have received funding from Pfizer.

The strategy, the summit, the submissions, the consumer group advocacy – 'It was like the perfect storm. It was all coming together,' Ms Brydon says. And this time, Lyrica was approved for subsidy. 'Absolutely, the two things are linked. Pfizer was very lucky we were doing what we were doing. The timing was exquisite, really,' says Ms Brydon. 'Self-interest drives these companies, and profit – let's not kid ourselves.'

Immediately after approval, Pfizer's selling campaign kicked into action. Between April and September 2012, Pfizer ran 91 'education events' for doctors relating to pain – almost four a week, according to University of Sydney researchers. Between April 2012 and September 2015, it would run 491 such events, at a cost of almost $3.8 million.

US studies have found that when a pharma company 'educates' doctors about a drug, they tend to prescribe more of it, and to do a worse job of making sure they're giving it for the right indications. 'We were seeing conferences being organised, bringing all the pain specialists in,' says pain doctor Tony Hall, one of the first in the country to prescribe subsidised Lyrica. 'GPs were prescribing it for every type of pain, not just nerve pain. That's an indication of just how widely Pfizer were promoting this medicine.'

In 2012, Pfizer paid a $US1 billion fine after the Department of Justice alleged it promoted four drugs, including Lyrica, for conditions that they were not medically indicated for – and paid doctors kickbacks for prescribing them.

Pfizer also sponsors major medical societies that represent doctors who prescribe Lyrica. One body that Pfizer supports is the Australian and New Zealand College of Anaesthetists (ANZCA), our peak body for pain medicine. Its most recent pain management evidence guidance is used by doctors around Australia to help people with acute pain. Pfizer put $25 000 toward the printing of that guidance document, and also supports the society's annual scientific meeting, annual refresher day course and the faculty's spring meeting. Including the printing costs, the college has received $199 470 from Pfizer in the last three years. The lead author of that guidance document has given Pfizer-sponsored speeches about Lyrica, although the company did not directly pay him to speak. The guidelines recommend pregabalin.

'An association between the college and the healthcare industry does not imply endorsement of products or services,' a spokeswoman for ANZCA told *The Age*. All funding was at arm's length. 'The college is meticulous in its approach to managing real or perceived conflicts of interest.'

Pfizer's network of sales representatives also swung into action. In LinkedIn posts, several Pfizer sales representatives brag about their successes selling Lyrica and getting it onto hospital 'formularies' – the hospital's stock of default drugs.

'I successfully achieved Lyrica formulary listings in the following hospitals by getting local Specialists to champion the listing,' said one. 'I know what it takes to get formulary of your product portfolio.'

That salesman also boasted that he specialised in 'GP surgery lunch meetings'. 'Lyrica PBS listing March 2012 with growth over 500 per cent,' he wrote.

In Australia, drug companies are not allowed to directly advertise drugs to consumers – a prohibition designed to stop money influencing treatment decisions. Instead, Pfizer rolled out a nerve-pain awareness campaign, suggesting to people with 'pain that won't go away' that it 'may be something called nerve pain'. 'If this is you, ask your doctor about nerve pain today,' the ads said. Pfizer's spokesman 'categorically denied' any link between the nerve pain awareness campaign and Lyrica.

In just six months in 2014, the awareness campaign had 24.1 million impressions, according to Pfizer's own data. Display advertising on the web reached another 2.1 million people. In 2012–13, doctors wrote 322 078 pregabalin scripts. In 2014–15, they wrote 2.69 million.

'They got a direct-to-consumer marketing program. Then you could fill in a form online to check your symptoms, and they'd say "You've got neuropathic back pain. Go see your doctor for some Lyrica",' says Professor Chris Maher.

That long, winding road from lobbying for approval through to 'educating' doctors and marketing to consumers eventually wound its way to Jacob Williams, who in 2017 had just left jail. One of the first things he did was to see his GP for a pregabalin prescription. Within a week of getting out, Mr Williams, 39, had a script for 300 milligrams – possibly for the back pain he had.

Like many addicts, Mr Williams abused pregabalin because of its ecstasy-like high, but also because it significantly increases the power of opiates, when they're consumed together. On 8 April 2022, his partner heard him gurgle, and then stop breathing. An autopsy later found a cocktail of drugs in his system, including potentially toxic levels of opiates and pregabalin. 'The Lyrica was supplied to him by a doctor,' his mother Jules Perrett told me. 'He would take so much he had no idea as to what day it was, let alone what he was doing. It did nothing for his nerve pain. This drug is dangerous when taken correctly and lethal when given to someone who suffers from substance abuse.'

In the emergency department of the Princess Alexandra Hospital in Brisbane, toxicologist Dr Katherine Isoardi sees pregabalin overdose cases come stumbling in – or wheeled in, comatose. Others are having seizures. More come every day, she says. 'It's got so much abuse potential. We're seeing people who are taking deliberate overdoses to harm themselves, but also people who are taking recreational doses to try to get high,' she says. Many people who come through show clear signs of mental health issues and self-harm, she says. Dr Isoardi cannot understand why they keep being given pregabalin prescriptions. 'A lot of people think of it as a safe option. And I don't think they appreciate you get tolerant, you get addicted, and it gets abused.'

When Pfizer launched Lyrica in Australia, it said the drug was likely not addictive because it did not bind to known opiate receptors. It's now clear that is wrong. Lyrica is addictive – and that addiction can be deadly. Almost half the pregabalin dispensed in Australia – two million scripts – is being used by just 15 per cent of the total group prescribed it, according to a study by the NSW Poisons Information Centre. This group of 86 000 appears to be abusing the drug. Three-quarters of these high-risk users were also prescribed opioids.

A Canadian study, published in August 2019, indicated pregabalin users had 1.7 times the risk of dying from an opioid overdose than opioid users alone – and high-dose users had 2.5 times the risk. Between 2004 and 2016, there were 1158 reports of 'intentional poisoning' – overdose – involving pregabalin made to the NSW Poisons Information Centre, increasing at 53.8 per cent a year. And ambulance attendances involving pregabalin jumped more than tenfold in Victoria from 2012, according to a paper published in November.

'It was initially promoted as having a low abuse potential,' says Nicholas Buckley, a professor of clinical pharmacology at the University of Sydney. 'But the warning signs were there almost from the beginning. It was reported to cause euphoria as a side effect – that's always a warning sign for abuse potential.'

A spokesman for Pfizer acknowledged 'post-marketing reports of substance misuse and abuse', but said the drug 'does not bind to known targets of abuse such as opiate receptors'. The drug had been demonstrated to be safe and effective, and was registered for use in more 130 countries, the spokesman said. They pointed to Health Department advice to doctors to vet patients for prior substance abuse before prescribing pregabalin. But this does not seem to be happening.

Experts said doctors seemed unaware of how addictive the drug could be, or that it can be abused. The study by the NSW Poisons Information Centre, led by Dr Rose Cairns, found that two-thirds of people who overdosed already had a pre-existing history of substance abuse when their doctors prescribed them pregabalin. Lyrica's listed side effects note that it doubles a patient's risk of suicidal thinking or behaviour versus a placebo to one case in every 530 people who use the medication. But almost 80 per cent of the overdose victims in Dr Cairns's study had been diagnosed with depression and 68 per cent had a history of suicidal thoughts. In 2018 the Health Department recorded seven suicide attempts, and six suicide deaths, suspected to be linked to pregabalin.

Of the first 50 people who went on pregabalin at one Gold Coast pain clinic in 2013 – just after the medicine had been added to the PBS – three reported the sudden onset of suicidal ideas. Tony Hall, a pharmacist at that clinic, had been giving out pregabalin for years – in much lower doses. 'It was either suicidal ideation or extreme anger. The doses Pfizer wanted us to give were completely wrong. We start them on 25 milligrams once a day, or then twice a day. Pfizer were telling us to start on 75 milligrams. Pain specialists have been saying for years we want a dose lower than 25 milligrams – this is a toxic medicine. It has lots of side effects.' When a patient complained to their GP about depression or suicidal ideation, the GP would often blame it on the pain and increase the pregabalin dose, Mr Hall says.

When Professor Chris Maher was running an independent trial on pregabalin at the University of Sydney, he almost had to stop over concerns for the safety of some of the volunteers. 'Some of the people in the trial said to us "I don't know what this medicine is, but … I've never had thoughts like that before",' he says. 'The GPs were sold the line by Pfizer that this is a safe medicine – get them off opioids and onto this. It's a horrible medicine. The side effects are confusion, drowsiness, disorientation, falling, suicidal ideation.'

Leona Solley, 55, describes a 'loss of empathy' which she links to the Lyrica her GP gave her for tingling and burning in her feet and fingertips. The drug made her feel foggy, disconnected from her husband and children. It sharply increased her anxiety. 'I got to the stage where I was thinking "Is it worth carrying on? I don't know if I can keep living like this",' she says. When she tried to quit, she suffered from what she says were withdrawal symptoms for six weeks. 'About five days after my last dosage, it was as though something was crawling under my skin and under my scalp. I had to cut all my fingernails because I was scratching myself so hard I was physically bleeding.'

There is now evidence pregabalin does not help even those people who have back pain. In a study published in the *New England Journal of Medicine* in 2017, University of Sydney Associate Professor Christine Lin and her colleagues showed pregabalin was no more effective than a placebo for treating sciatica (Pfizer disputes those results). 'It does not work,' Professor Lin says. 'And we know it has side effects.'

The story of Lyrica is deeply troubling, but not in any way surprising. Lyrica was marketed as a replacement for opioids, but its story in fact mirrors that of opioids. Lyrica slots into place in a long, long cycle: first we embrace opioids, then we pay the price, then we forget those lessons and return to our blissful, deadly embrace.

'I was virtually numb. It got to the stage where nothing really mattered,' Stuart Leamer told the ABC in 2020. Prescribed codeine in the mid-1990s after injuring his back while helping a friend build a house, Mr Leamer quickly worked his way up: first OxyContin and then morphine. He would stay on the drugs for more than two decades – a new prescription written every month for him by his doctor. 'I missed kids' birthdays, I missed grandkids' birthdays, fishing, going out in the garden,' he said. At his lowest point, he considered suicide.

It all began in Tasmania ...

You've likely read something of the opioid crisis that first engulfed America before spreading around the western world. You may not know that the story of opioids, to a great extent, is a story about back pain – and it's one that starts right here, in Tasmania.

If you were to venture there, passing the sheep farmers in battered LandCruisers and the hobby farmers in shining Teslas, you'd find fields and fields of poppies, *Papaver somniferum*, flowers gently fluttering in the breeze. But these aren't just any poppies.

In 1994, chemists at a Johnson & Johnson subsidiary called Tasmanian Alkaloids worked out how to tweak the poppy plant, changing its chemical structure so the plant naturally produced much higher levels of thebaine, one chemical precursor for making the powerful designer opioid oxycodone, reports Peter Smith in the *Pacific Standard*.[1] The company called this new variety 'Norman'; soon, these 'super-poppies' grew in fields and paddocks across the island – many hung with signs that read 'Poison'.[2]

The US government had strong rules governing the importation of narcotic raw materials like morphine, designed to limit the ability of pharmaceutical companies to flood the market with dangerous opioids. But in 2000 they decided these rules did not apply to thebaine, perhaps because of claims it was less prone to abuse.[3] The companies could import as much of it as they wanted. The Hobart *Mercury* heralded it as an 'export coup'. And with 'Norman', Johnson & Johnson was able to make the chemical in greater quantities at less than half the cost. Tasmanian Alkaloids started shipping the chemicals to America. Unknown and untracked by almost anyone, Tasmania soon emerged as the world's leading supplier of legal opioids, Peter Smith writes in *Pacific Standard*. By 2011 it was supplying about 80 per cent of the world's oxycodone raw materials. The company's thebaine was in such high demand it was paying local Tasmanian farmers megabucks – some even received BMWs and Mercedes-Benzes – to rip out existing crops and replace them with poppies.

After Tasmania's role in the crisis became known, many journalists went down and sought out the poppy farmers to ask if they felt any guilt. They said they did not.[4] They were just growing the poppies and shipping them away. It was America's pharma companies who were truly at fault, they said.

That may be true. But Tasmania is still paying the price: Australia's poorest state is also the country's epicentre for opioids, writes Kristen Gelineau in the *Australian Financial Review*.[6] It now has the nation's highest rate of opioid packs sold per person. One region of the state hands out 110 000 prescriptions for 100 000 people.

The 'Norman' poppies were harvested and shipped to manufacturing facilities, where the milky white liquid in seed capsules was transformed into opioids – principally oxycodone.

Opioids like oxycodone bind to opioid receptors located in the brain and spinal cord, both blocking pain signals from other parts of the body[5] and releasing large amounts of the pleasure neurotransmitter dopamine – the same chemical released when we do things our brain wants to encourage, like eating or having sex. Since antiquity, humans have been looking to extract more and more powerful highs from the poppy – first opium, and then morphine, and then heroin, each magnitudes more powerful than the last. OxyContin was the next point of that cycle: a partially synthetic superpowered shot.

OxyContin's active ingredient is oxycodone, which has been in use in America since the beginning of the 21st century. But the drug's key technological innovation was a slow-release mechanism, which could provide a dozen hours of pain relief.

OxyContin was the creation of Purdue Pharma. It would initially tout the new drug as a powerful painkiller with almost no risk of addiction – much safer, in fact, than other opioids.[7] Originally it was marketed for short-term and extremely painful conditions like end-stage cancer, pain relief after surgery, and AIDS.

Opioids move in cycles: seduction, horror, forgetfulness, seduction. They first hit the pharmaceutical market in the mid-1850s, when chemists learnt to isolate a key active ingredient, morphine – named after Morpheus, the god of dreams.[8] Abuse, addiction and death soon followed, so chemists made efforts to develop a safer, non-addictive opioid. In 1898 a new, purportedly addiction- and abuse-free drug was synthesised: heroin. Bayer sold it as a cough remedy. Within years it was being abused on the street, and addicts were soon beating down the doors of hospitals, seeking their fix.[9] Doctors, horrified, swore off the lure of the poppy.

But in the 1980s and 1990s, the cycle was starting to run the other way. Pain was increasingly becoming seen as a problem in its own right, something that needed treatment.

US states started to pass laws giving doctors more freedom to prescribe controlled substances for intractable pain. In 1995, the American Pain Society launched a new campaign calling for doctors to recognise pain as a 'fifth vital sign'. Unfortunately, unlike heart rate and blood pressure, pain is a subjective experience – opening the way for addicted patients to demand more and more painkillers. Australia followed suit, approving opioids for treating non-cancer pain in the year 2000, and adding a government subsidy on top.[10]

Meanwhile, Purdue had something to sell. Purdue was owned by members of the Sackler family. The family's patriarch Arthur – described by one journalist as the Don Draper of pharmaceutical marketing – was a pioneer in a very specialised type of ad.[11] Rather than targeting patients with ads – although he did that too – Sackler's real genius was to realise you needed to sell to doctors too. 'He recognised that selling new drugs requires a seduction of not just the patient,' wrote Patrick Keefe in the *New Yorker*, 'but the doctor who writes the prescription.'

To do that, Arthur – who died several years before the launch of OxyContin – had learnt you needed some level of scientific credibility.[12] That meant finding and amplifying scientific papers – ones that said what you wanted them to say.

In 1980, two doctors in Boston, Jane Porter and Hershel Jick, penned a short letter on addiction to the *New England Journal of Medicine*.[13] Of 11 882 patients given opioids at their Boston hospital, the doctors wrote, there were just four cases of addiction. This 'study' would go on to become the basis of the Sacklers' new wave of opioids, and the centre of Purdue's marketing strategy. Purdue's marketing told doctors it demonstrated that less than 1 per cent of people given opioids become addicted. But it was no study – just a five-sentence letter to the editor, merely 101 words long. No experiments were done; there's no detail about how the finding was arrived at. That single letter has now been cited more than 608 times.

To amplify the message, the Sacklers found highly respected doctors and paid them to speak for Purdue, espousing the benefits of their products. Who were in the audience? Doctors from across the country, flown in for free to listen to the spiel – and then enjoy the free buffet afterwards.

The company ran more than 40 pain management and speaker training conferences at all-expenses-paid resorts across America between 1996 and 2001, recruiting and training more than 5000 doctors, nurses and pharmacists for its 'speaker bureau'. It showered doctors with free hats, stuffed toys and music CDs (*Get in the swing with OxyContin*), writes journalist Beth Macy in her chronicle of the scandal, *Dopesick*. To get patients hooked, it offered coupons for a free month's supply. Marketing centred on that key claim from Porter and Jick's little letter that less than 1 per cent of all users of OxyContin became addicted. It trained its sales staff to push that message. The drug went on to become a blockbuster for Purdue: revenue shot from US$48 million in 1996 to $3.1 billion in 2010.

These ideas even infiltrated medical schools. '[As a medical student] we were told that if someone has legitimate pain, they could not develop addiction. We now know that's absolutely untrue,' says Professor Suzanne Nielsen, a pharmaceutical researcher and deputy director of the Monash Addiction Research Centre.

Opioids were initially marketed for 'acute end-of-life pain' and the pain that comes from cancer – extreme, intractable pain, where the doctor's goal is simply to give relief. But those pains are a small market, relatively speaking. And nearly everyone has back pain. Before OxyContin, people with serious pain were typically given simple painkillers or low-dose opioids. The sales documents of Purdue show that it relentlessly targeted people with back pain, as well as the family doctors who both typically saw these cases and weren't specialists in treating pain.

One promotional video course featured a series of hypothetical patients, including construction worker Johnny Sullivan, who told the audience how OxyContin had eased his back pain. He later became addicted to the drug. In 2008 he apparently blacked out, rolled his truck, and died.

'Back pain was a target because it's so common, and even if you ran a campaign for chronic pain, you still captured back pain as it's the most common form of chronic pain,' says Chris Maher.

US insurance data suggests opioids are the most-prescribed class of drug for back pain; more than half of regular opioid users report they suffer from back pain.[14] In Australia, almost 20 per cent of patients with back pain will be given opioids; two-thirds of patients who turn up at hospital with back pain get a script.

Just two years after OxyContin went on sale in America, Perdue established an Australian subsidiary: Mundi-pharma. Australia bans the sort of direct-to-consumer drug advertising seen in America, but there's nothing to prohibit drug companies here advertising to doctors.

That's exactly what Mundipharma did, an investigation by my colleague Farrah Tomazin revealed. The company held product launch meetings over three-course dinners, spent tens of thousands of dollars sponsoring conferences, and ran a pain management master class which almost 5000 medical professionals have taken.

The company invited Australian doctors to a conference in Italy for the International Association for the Study of Pain, wining and dining Australian doctors in Milan, spent $8200 on a drinks-and-canapes 'product launch meeting' for pharmacists, and ran an all-expenses-paid 'pain masterclass' for GPs at a luxury hotel in Brisbane, at a cost of $128 000.[15]

Mundipharma distributed a brochure advertising its new opioid Targin – a reformulation containing oxycodone and naloxone, a drug that quells opioid-induced constipation. The brochure glibly claimed strong slow-release opioids, like oxycodone, were less likely to cause addiction than weak instant-hit versions – the same false claim Purdue had used to defend OxyContin. The company ended up paying a $302 400 fine for false advertising.

Oxycodone did not succeed because it was any better than competing opioids – it wasn't.[16] It succeeded because of the way it was sold. In just a few years, these advertising campaigns would help convert so many people to opioids that it created a subset industry for laxatives – also sold by Perdue – to relieve opioid-caused constipation.[17]

Rustie Lastam started taking them at 16 to treat chronic back pain. During her pregnancy, the La Trobe Valley mother was swallowing nine high-dose tablets a day. Her child emerged from the womb addicted; she remembers the wailing of her infant son as he went through withdrawal. 'If only they knew what addiction did to people, how really it affects us to the very core of who we are,' she told the Associated Press's Kristen Gelineau. 'And there they are, making all this money off the back of my broken life.'

Treatment at hospitals and surgeries also played a role. Spine surgery, out of all musculoskeletal surgeries, has the highest rate of persistent opioid use, and anterior lumbar interbody fusion is number one in spine surgeries.

Do the opioids work? There is now high-quality evidence that they do not. A trial of 240 patients with back and knee pain, published in *JAMA* in 2018,[18] randomised them between 12 months of opioid therapy and 12 months of taking paracetamol. After 12 months there were no differences in actual recovery – and the paracetamol group were in much *less* pain.

Why might this be? Opioids seem to be an extraordinarily powerful painkiller. Meet *opioid-induced hyperalgesia*. At high doses, for long enough, opioids actually mess with the central nervous system and make the nerves more sensitive to pain. Opioids work because they mimic natural painkillers the body releases when it's in pain. But the body *needs* pain to survive – we need to yank our hand away from a hot stove, for example. It seems our bodies have evolved mechanisms, when exposed to too much opioid, to ramp up pain, to make sure we take notice. If your back's sore and you're hooked on opioids, its entirely possible your painkiller is actually making your pain worse.

Dad had his own brush with opioids. When he checked

into a pain clinic – this one had him rubbing lanolin into his hamstrings every day – they doped him up. Hard. Sixty milligrams of OxyContin a day (a formula so strong it's no longer sold in Australia), plus the sedative Valium. No wonder he barely remembers anything from his time at the clinic.

He inevitably got hooked, although not as seriously as a full-blown addict. 'I was concerned I would never live without them,' he says. As he says it, my mind flashes to the cupboards in his bedroom, which used to overflow with small zip-lock bags filled with pills. Mum would beg him to throw them out – 'They must be expired by now!' – but he never would.

At the peak of the problem, Dad says, his life became very strange and troubled. 'I had a few weeks of intermittent nightmares, and was very restless, and at one stage drove to Horsham and ended up in a hotel getting a massage by a man with a blue singlet, bulging biceps, boots and a beard, but a gentle smile,' Dad says. 'I couldn't work out how I got there or why he was there. The receptionist told me later that when I arrived she thought I was coming down off drugs and needed some help. Which I got.'

After his back surgery appeared to relieve the pain, he managed to kick the pill habit – although he'd carry the pills with him for a decade more. Only last year he went on his first trip without them, he tells me.

Purdue would plead for years it did not know about OxyContin's addictive properties. But evidence, much of it from discovery in lawsuits, has emerged showing this is wrong. Purdue knew. A company-funded study from 1999 on patients using OxyContin for headaches found

13 per cent of users became addicted, Patrick Radden Keefe discovered.

Ultimately, perhaps one person in every ten who take opioids for chronic pain will end up either addicted or dependent. The problem for anyone thinking of taking them, says Suzanne Nielsen, is that 'we're not actually very good at predicting who might develop dependence.' To begin an unwisely prescribed course of opioids is to play Russian roulette with addiction.

Why? A certain group of people will experience a euphoric bliss when they use opioids. Some of that is genetic, but some of it is environmental as well; the ability to escape daily life is most attractive for those who have a life they want to leave. Most people who become addicted will remain addicted for life. People who do manage to break the addiction are often left with permanent mental and physical damage.

More than 80 000 Americans died in 2021 from opioid overdose – up more than 10 000 from a year before. In Australia, at least three people die from opioid harm every day, while another 150 are hospitalised.

Decades since OxyContin was first approved, the wheel is starting to turn. Lawsuits in multiple US states have crippled Purdue; more are expected. Regulators have cracked down, forcing the industry to move to abuse-resistant formulations and setting up databases to watch for doctor shopping. In Australia, you can't even buy Panadeine Forte over the counter any more. We are once again awake to opioids' terrible power.

As decades of healthcare warnings and restrictions led tobacco use to fall in the western world, tobacco companies pivoted to the underdeveloped east and south. And so it now is with opioids; Mundipharma are pushing into new markets, places where doctors and regulators are not yet awake to the danger. In Brazil and China, they are reusing the same old tactics: sales pitches to doctors designed to overcome their fear of opioids.

'We're only just getting started,' Mundipharma's promotional videos declare.

Paracetamol does not help back pain

What about something safer?

For a long time, paracetamol was the default recommendation for anyone with back pain. Cheap, harmless, and available in the supermarket. Why not try it? But that's no longer the thinking from leading back pain experts.

In 2015 a team of Australian researchers led by Gustavo Machado conducted a meta-analysis on just how well the pills actually worked for pain. They concluded with high confidence that paracetamol simply does not work for back pain any better than a placebo. 'Millions of Australians are taking drugs that not only don't work very well, they're causing harm,' Machado told *The Age*.

And paracetamol's reputation for safety has taken a battering. It's surprisingly easy to overdose – a person taking the drug to the maximum recommendation would end up ingesting 4 grams over 24 hours, and just 5 grams of the drug can cause liver complications, with harm increasing as you get into higher numbers. Take a few extra pills, or forget another medicine you're on *also* has paracetamol in it, and you're quickly into the danger zone. That's part of the reason why paracetamol is the number one drug Australia's poison control centres get calls about; more than 95 000 people were hospitalised from an overdose between 2007 and 2017 (about three-quarters of those cases were intentional overdoses), and more than 200 people died. Those risks showed up in Machado's data. People using the drug to treat back pain were nearly four times more likely to have abnormalities show up on liver function tests.

'For anti-inflammatories like ibuprofen, the story is different,' Machado says. Here, the data indicates they do help with back pain – but only a little. 'The effect is small and may not be considered important by patients,' he says. 'At the moment, there aren't many options. We know paracetamol doesn't work. We know ibuprofen works, but the effect is quite small. We know the harms of opioids outweigh the benefits.'

8   Spinal surgery

Shannon Noll grew up in Tullibigeal and Condobolin, a pair of tiny towns surrounded by endless farms in central New South Wales. He spent the first 20 years of his life working on the 4500-acre family farm. After a long day, he and his brothers would toss guitars in the back of the family ute and drive out to play at whichever pub would have them.

Farming in Australia isn't easy. A run of bad luck can quickly pile up and overwhelm. The long drought at the turn of the century pushed the Nolls' farm deep into debt. Then Shannon's father was killed in a farm accident. The brothers tried to farm their way out, but the weather refused to relent. Up to their eyeballs in debt, they needed some luck.

That luck arrived in the form of reality television imported from the UK: *Australian Idol*. Hundreds of thousands of viewers tuned in. And there was Shannon. White shirt, soul patch on his chin, nervous. For the audition he chose 'Hold me in your arms', by the Southern Sons.

> So my love, hold me in your arms
> Time moves without us, this room will be untouched
> We're safe beneath the truth now
> Both safe within this love

The panel of judges looked stunned. 'We have just discovered,' Marcia Hines told him, shaking her head, 'a voice.' From there, Noll's star would rapidly ascend into the firmament. Runner-up in the competition, followed by two number-one albums and three chart-topping singles. His luck, and his family's luck, had finally turned.

But while Noll's star was rising, his back was starting to trouble him. 'I had bad posture on the farm, doing bits and pieces of farm work and shearing, and that was where it started,' he tells me. 'Dad had a crook back. Mum's brothers as well. Just lifting stuff off the ground with the wrong posture was where it all started.'

Noll is a pin-up boy for some of the problems and risks that go with spinal surgery. The surgeries – which range from a simple decompression to a multi-level fusion of several vertebrae, right up to inserting an artificial disc – are as popular as they are expensive. Yet there are serious questions about how well several surgical options for back pain work, with many major expert groups warning against having one at all. At first, Noll put up with the pain and got on with his life. He took that back, sore and stiff and aching, on tour around Australia and the world. And then something snapped – on *Dancing with the Stars*.

'It's so embarrassing,' says Noll. 'I was supposed to catch my partner from the side. And I wasn't ready, and she launched, and I just caught her – and it ripped it sideways.' 'It' was one of Noll's spinal discs. Noll tells me the impact from the catch compressed his spine, the force overwhelming one of his spinal discs, blowing a hole in the side and squeezing the disc's innards out into his spinal canal. In severe pain, he pulled out of rehearsals. But he had a gig booked for the next day, and there was no disappointing the fans. He flew up, and then back to Melbourne for Sunday's main show – *Dancing* was filmed live in front of a studio audience.

Somehow, Noll managed to do the show. He woke up on Monday in agony. 'I couldn't move. I'd never had pain like that before.' The pain ran all the way down the right side of his back, through his buttocks, and into his leg, filling the limb with pins and needles. 'I was going "I have to get to hospital – quick".'

An ambulance ran Noll to the nearest emergency department, where a doctor told him he'd need a discectomy, also known as decompression surgery. Noll's herniated disc was pressing on nerves in his spine, likely including his sciatic nerve, which was causing the leg pain. The surgeon made a cut between the vertebrae and carefully fished out the ejected disc material pressing on the nerve. The operation was a partial success, Noll says. The serious, acute pain went away. In its place came creeping chronic back pain. 'You get up in the morning and you're f----d putting your socks on. That was from 2012. You're stiff and sore all the time,' he tells me. His right foot was oddly disobedient – not all the time, but every so often he'd tell it to go here and it would go there and Noll would trip.

'A couple days after the operation, I woke up in the morning with blood all through the sheets. I'd had pins and needles in my toe, had been scratching it, couldn't feel it, and had scratched through the skin and bled all over the sheets,' Noll says.

After I interviewed Noll, the newspaper sent photographer Edwina Pickles down to Lilli Pilli Point on Sydney's glittering coastline to get a snap. The pictures are amazing.

Noll, who has clearly done this before, stands on the shore, jaw jutting, dog tags hanging on muscled chest, unbuttoned white dress shirt flapping in the breeze, a true rock star.

Down the front of his abdomen, cutting vertically through his belly button: a long, dark scar.

Noll's decompression surgery fixed his acute pain. But it left him with chronic, long-term lower back pain. To deal with the pain, Noll turned to the gym: four to five sessions a week, focusing on his core strength. You can see that hard work in the photos. He spoke to many people, he says, who'd also struggled with back pain. After training their core and building muscular strength, they told him, the pain went away. 'But I don't know,' Noll sighs heavily, a bit forlorn. 'I don't know what I was doing. There was no sign that was ever going to work out for me. No matter what I did it was still going to be there, hurtin'.' With the gym not helping, Noll turned to medicine. He saw surgeon after surgeon in the hope that one of them would be able to offer him relief.

They all took one look at his scan and told him he needed a spinal fusion. 'Nuh uh,' says Noll. 'I said I wasn't having one, because I'd heard so many horror stories about it.' Noll tried anti-inflammatory injections. But they were only a short-term fix. Eventually, an exhausted Noll ended up where he did not want to be – on a surgeon's table.

His surgeon told him his spine was so degenerated his vertebrae had started fusing. 'So if we do a fusion, we're just speeding up the process,' Noll recalls saying. 'He said "You might be pain free in four years, or ten years", if I did not have the fusion.' The other option Noll was offered was opioids. He wasn't doing that. He'd seen too many people lose their way on the powerful drugs. 'You just end up walking around like a zombie.'

Fusion seemed like the best of a bad bunch of options. Noll, weary of fighting what felt like a losing battle with his back, agreed to the surgery. A few days later, a nurse swabbed his arm, an IV line was slid beneath the flesh, and everything turned black. The surgeon performed a fusion, and slid in an artificial disc – a so-called 'hybrid' procedure for multiple levels of joint pain. 'I came out of the operation,' says Noll, 'and just started *screaming* with the pain. The doctor said it went absolutely swimmingly, couldn't have gone better. He said "You've had your spine cut in half, that's why it hurts".'

It took me a few weeks to get Noll's surgeon on the phone. Based at a private hospital in an inner suburb, he's a very busy man. But I was keen to talk to him. I wanted to understand his thinking: why use a fusion? And what was really causing Noll's pain?

'When I saw him,' the surgeon tells me, 'he was really struggling.' Once you lose a bit of jelly from inside a disc, you don't get it back, he said. 'The damage is done. But you keep using it, and you start having what we call discogenic low back pain – pain coming from the disc.'

Sometimes when a disc is injured, the body's natural healing methods can cause problems by laying down tiny new nerves in the disc, the surgeon says. 'This is why you have patients with bad discs, and it does not cause pain. But some with bad discs, it causes pain all the time – because they have nerves growing into it.' Without its supportive inner filling, Noll's disc was already 'starting to fuse to the surrounding vertebrae'.

'That's why, if you look at old people, they hunch over. Because their discs are losing water. And the discs are fusing together. We do a fusion because that's what nature is trying to do.' He confirmed that he did add an artificial disc to Noll's spine as well as perform a fusion. 'I have to either put in an artificial disc – that's what we did – or we fuse it, because that's what nature's trying to do,' he says.

Was there anything Noll could have done to avoid having his spine fused and disc replaced, I asked? The surgeon pondered that for a while. 'Shannon was fit, he was trying his best. I think he's just been unlucky,' he eventually told me. 'There's nothing the poor guy could have done differently.'

Could this be true? Was Noll simply destined for a spinal fusion the moment he lifted his dance partner? Perhaps. But in most cases, other experts told me, the evidence simply does not support the use of spinal fusion for treating chronic low back pain.

Spinal fusion joins two vertebrae, permanently. The idea is to weld together the vertebrae and encourage them to grow into a single, strong bone. The operation is principally designed to improve stability in the spine, and is typically used when surgeons are worried about spinal degeneration.[1]

The hard surface of the vertebrae is shaved away, and rods and screws, or plates and pins (there are lots of different ways of doing it), are inserted to join the bones together. Typically, something is placed in between to encourage the bones to fuse – often bone drilled from the patient's hip, that gets placed into a food processor and ground into a fine pulp.

Spinal fusions rarely work for back pain

Spinal fusion started with the best of intentions. The procedure came out of attempts to deal with spinal fractures and spinal tuberculosis.[2] The operation works in these cases, and in many cases is life-saving. But over time, fusion's use has dramatically expanded. What started out as a treatment for a curved spine is now routinely offered for back pain and degenerative disc disease. Conditions which – sadly – they often don't work for. 'You can't unbugger a buggered back by rebuggering it,' writes spinal surgeon Bruce McPhee. 'Often surgeons don't know when not to operate or when to stop operating. When not to operate is the greatest test for a spinal surgeon.'

Shortly before he planned to retire, Brisbane-based neurosurgeon Leigh Atkinson penned an article for an academic journal lifting the lid on the truth about spinal fusions for back pain: *they rarely worked*, and we were doing way too many of them.[3] He told me he was deluged with phone calls – from surgeons complaining and from patients saying he'd hit the nail on the head. He stands by what he wrote.

There were six core ways of doing a spinal fusion today, he told me. Why? 'If there are six different ways, it means there's nothing they're confident will work,' Dr Atkinson said.

It was also driven by a rapid expansion in the different types of implantable metal for sale; surgeons, like anyone, became very excited at the site of a shiny new toy, and itched to try them out in their patients. Some surgeons even opt for more technically challenging fusions because they like the challenge. 'It's like how sailors like to sail in dangerous seas, even though it's dangerous,' Atkinson told me. 'And a lot of surgeons want to operate. That's what they're there for. A lot of them have a lot of belief in their own capacity. It's easier to talk a patient into an operation than talk one out of an operation – most people want some sort of cure.'

Now, there are good reasons for doing a spinal fusion. Malignancy, infection, fracture, says Patrick Owen, a researcher who studies the disc at Deakin University's Institute for Physical Activity and Nutrition. But most people – perhaps 99 per cent of everyone with back pain – don't have those specific, diagnosable problems. They just have back pain. And the published scientific evidence suggests Atkinson's anecdote is, if anything, too kind on spinal fusions and surgery for back pain in general.

Cochrane reviewed the evidence for spinal fusion for stenosis – narrowing of the spinal canal, a common reason for fusion – in 2016, and concluded *there was no evidence surgery was superior to conservative care*, and that conservative care was much safer.[4]

Harris, Maher and Buchbinder did their own review of the evidence for spinal fusions for low back pain and degenerative disc disease in 2018.[5] They concluded there was simply no evidence fusion worked any better than conservative care – think physio rehab – for low back pain caused by degenerated discs. And, again, surgery was less safe: they estimated the surgical complication rate at 16 per cent.

Two new Australian studies put those numbers into real world context. The first study looked at 874 injured Victorian workers who received a spinal fusion between 2008 and

2016.[6] Overall, the surgery led to only an 8 per cent increase in the number of people with substantial work capacity, and 77 people who were working before the operation were *not* working two years after the surgery.

The second study, looking at injured NSW workers who'd had spine surgery, found even more dismal outcomes – and substantial harms.[7] After a spinal fusion, just 19 per cent had returned to work within two years. Almost one in five patients needed a second spine surgery within two years of the first operation, with some needing up to five reoperations.

So bad were its outcomes, WorkSafe Victoria set up panels of surgeons to review proposed spinal fusions. Over the 18 months to December 2019, the panel rejected almost half of the fusions proposed by outside surgeons, suggesting at least some surgeons are far too trigger-happy when it comes to an expensive surgery with little chance of success. Many surgeons seem blind to that evidence, Chris Maher says. 'They believe in it. It's like going to Hillsong [Church]. They're telling us: I know in my patients this works.' But, says Maher, they just don't.

Ashish Diwan, the spine surgeon we met earlier, tells me he does perform spinal fusions for people with back pain who've tried everything else. When I ask him if they work, his answer is considered and nuanced. 'I don't know,' he says. 'Will I do it? Yes, and I do. When patients come and ask me would I get it done for myself, I tell them: *no*. But they say they're suffering – so I say, if you feel I should do it then I will do it.'

'Do all of them get better? No. Sixty per cent are very grateful. Twenty per cent are worse off, but don't tell that to me. But they are still grateful to me – it was their choice to get it done. And another 20 per cent are just the same.'

Maree Rivero – we met her earlier, when her GP nicked her spinal cord while trying to administer an epidural – eventually ended up receiving a spinal fusion, although there were a few more twists to her story before she got there.

Nothing else worked to treat the pain, which was like a knife in the back, she tells me. She had lower back pain but no leg pain. Doctors imaged her spine and told her she had severe disc degeneration. She tried everything: Pilates, yoga, chiropractic, massage, floating in a small pool of magnesium-heavy water. Her pain got worse.

She, like Noll, had become trapped in the back pain spiral. She, like Noll, eventually and in desperation ended up in front of a spine surgeon.

Her surgeon was reluctant to operate. She had no leg pain, which meant there was no evidence the discs were putting pressure on her spinal nerves. She was sent home.

'On the way home from the surgeon, my L5 disc blew – it exploded,' says Rivero.' She offers to send me a picture. 'It was sitting on my spinal cord. I couldn't walk.'

She contacted her existing surgeon who ordered immediate scans, as now she had severe leg pain. Her surgeon reviewed these scans and advised her to get to Melbourne immediately. A new surgeon reviewed her scans at a Repatriation hospital; he agreed she needed immediate surgery and was able to get her admitted to another hospital that same day. Her existing surgeon came to see her in hospital to conduct the surgery. He would fuse her, he offered. But how many levels did she want, he asked, pointing out that two discs showed signs of degeneration.

She chose to have both done, reasoning she'd just need another fusion at a later time.

'The surgery itself went really well,' Rivero says. 'It was very, very painful. I don't think there's anything on planet Earth that will prepare you for when those drugs wear off. When they first got me on my feet, I nearly vomited on the nurse in pain.'

Rivero was sent home within a few days, with instructions to spend as much time on her feet as possible. A few days later, she started to feel unwell. She ran a fever. She felt shaky. The pain at her surgical site went from horrible to horrific to unbearable.

She was taken back to hospital, where doctors soon discovered she'd contracted an antibiotic-resistant surgical infection in the site. She was airlifted to a major hospital in Melbourne, where another set of doctors reopened her spine to scrub the infection out.

Rivero survived, somehow. She's back walking, back going to the gym. Her fusion is fusing nicely. But she's not back-pain free.

'I'm exercising, I'm fit and healthy,' says Rivero. 'I have my life back. But I think I will always have lower back pain.'

In October 2010, Barry Espinos booked himself in to see a neurosurgeon. Espinos was 55, and running a sand supply business in Geraldton, Western Australia, that he'd painstakingly built up from scratch so that it could employ his brothers and his wife. He had dropped out of school at about 14, but discovered a penchant for and a joy in working on machines – earthmovers, loaders, trucks. When his father fell ill, he bought a plane, built an airstrip and got a pilot's licence, all so he could fly down to see him and Espinos's growing brood of grandchildren in Perth on weekends.

In 2009, Espinos was driving a grader – a heavy-duty machine that uses a huge blade to level asphalt or gravel roads – when it flipped on the edge of a levee. Espinos bailed out in the nick of time, avoiding being crushed by the huge machine, but landed hard on his backside.

He kept working, and didn't think too much of the fall. But over time, he developed a nagging pain in his back and leg that wouldn't go away. Rather than referring him to a physiotherapist, his GP sent him straight off for facet joint injections – which did not work.

Still struggling with his back, Espinos got a tip from a friend about a local spine surgeon. He and his wife visited the surgeon's office together, and the prognosis was good: after the operation he'd be 80 per cent better, court documents say he was told. At this stage, he was still working.

Espinos went under on the surgeon's table a month later. But the surgeon fused the wrong level. Espinos woke up in pain, which only got worse – much worse than it was before the operation. Heavily dosed on pain pills, the hardworking, intelligent grandfather soon found himself in a mess. When he next saw his surgeon, Espinos was in a wheelchair. Despite that, the surgeon told him the surgery had gone well, Espinos recalled.

Eventually, the surgeon agreed to have another go, opening him up a month later. But the tissue had become infected, the surgeon discovered. That would need to be treated first.

After that was cleared, two months later, Espinos again went under. This time the surgeon fused the right level, while also replacing screws on the level he had mistakenly fused. When Espinos woke up, the pain was somehow *worse* – so bad he thought the surgeon had left something inside his back when he sewed him up. A CT scan showed both the screws had been misplaced, one sticking laterally out of the spine and the other penetrating Espinos's spinal cord. Again, another surgery was performed to remove and replace both screws; by this point Espinos could not walk. This also did not work, and so Espinos had another surgery – to repair the spine and implant a spinal cord stimulator. He sold his beloved aircraft, he told the court, because his head was in such a mess and he 'did not want to hurt anybody'. He had to close his business. He struggled to drive or walk even short distances. He couldn't help his wife around the house. He couldn't play with his grandchildren.

'In total, Mr Espinos has undergone eight spinal operations,' wrote the judge in the eventual, inevitable medical negligence lawsuit. 'The consequences of all of this for Mr Espinos have been disastrous.' The court eventually awarded him $4.8 million in compensation.

From what we know of Noll's story, a discectomy might seem to be the right course of action. The evidence suggests these operations are highly effective surgeries in people in serious pain – think hospitalisation – caused by an exploded disc putting pressure on a sensitive spinal nerve. Cochrane's reviewers found in the right patients it substantially beat conservative treatment over the short term.

However, over the long term, patients who had surgery did no better than those who did not. The surgery provided immediate pain relief, but there is no strong evidence it beat doing nothing – and leaving the body to heal – over the long term.

Why? Because 90 per cent of bad sciatica attacks will settle without surgery if you leave them. In most cases, a ruptured disc can pull itself back together.

'There are several big studies that show a resolution rate of between 70 to 90 per cent of most disc herniations, over a period of about three months. This includes everyone: people with minor and more severe symptoms,' says Dr Mike Selby, a spine surgeon based in Adelaide. 'Never rush the decision for surgery.'

The indications for surgery tend to be when something is seriously wrong. If the nerve is so compressed it is causing weakness, like a dropped foot or difficulty standing, there is a good case for going in quickly before the nerve is permanently damaged. 'You cannot guarantee that will recover even if the disc resolves with time, because that process may take too long,' he says.

It's possible Noll's injury might have settled, but given the extreme pain he was in – pain so bad he couldn't walk – surgery seems like an evidence-based option. But unfortunately it only worked partially for Noll. And here we get into the problems with taking the surgical path.

'Chronic pain is a pretty common outcome for a discectomy,' says Chris Maher. 'There are people who have the surgery and their leg pain gets better, but they still have back pain. And the problem then becomes when they think they need another surgery to fix up the back pain. And that's when you're in an evidence-free zone: people start doing things like fusions and spinal cord stimulators.'

As the evidence spinal fusion works so poorly for lower back pain has started to accumulate, governments have come under increasing pressure to act. The Australian government tried to fix the problem. They failed – and the reasons why are instructive about our whole back pain system.

In 2015, concerns around spinal fusion costs were coming to a head. Private health insurers were ramping up pressure on the government to take action. Bupa private health insurance managing director Dr Dwayne Crombie described the operation as 'a waste of time', while Private Healthcare Australia head Rachel David told *The Australian* 'we know that probably only around 20 patients out of every 100 who get spinal fusion surgery are helped by it. But it gets a lot of funding … and doctors will just come back and say we don't know which 20 per cent benefit, so they're continuing to operate on people.' Some insurers even dropped spinal fusion coverage – drawing outrage from doctors.

The federal government decided something needed to be done: a root-and-branch review of the entire Medicare system.

Meanwhile, a second separate process was underway. Choosing Wisely, a campaign targeting medical waste and dodgy treatments, was launched in the same year by NPS MedicineWise, the government-funded organisation charged with incorporating evidence into healthcare. From the start, both campaigns had spinal fusion in their sights, one concerned about money and the other about patient outcomes.

In 2018, Choosing Wisely issued strong guidelines from the Australian and New Zealand College of Anaesthetists' Faculty of Pain Medicine: *do not refer anyone with low back pain for spinal fusion.*

With the evidence behind them, the federal government announced later that year it would ban surgeons for billing Medicare for spinal fusions to treat uncomplicated chronic low back pain – the very indication, as we've seen, it works so poorly for. To deal with private insurance, the government proposed changes meaning spinal fusion would only be covered by the most expensive tier of insurance.

The lobbying started almost immediately. Gold Coast orthopaedic surgeon Associate Professor Matthew Scott-Young told my colleague Lucy Stone the proposed changes would leave people in pain, or push them toward less-evidence-based treatments. Dr Marc Coughlan, a Sydney-based neurosurgeon, was quoted in the same article worrying about the spines of young people. 'It would potentially impact the lives of thousands of patients who would be precluded from having spinal fusions because of the high costs,' he said. 'Many of these people are younger patients with spinal conditions impacting on their ability to walk, work and remain productive in the workforce.'

Then the Australian Medical Association made an extra-ordinary submission to the government claiming that it had not been consulted about the changes. A survey of its members contained a range of pissed-off responses from surgeons, who compared the – evidence-based – guidelines to refrain from fusion for low-back pain to 'medical negligence'.

The survey gives us a great insight into the mindset of some surgeons. One noted that surgery for back pain had an important place in treating 'failed previous back surgery'. Another, in defending surgery, wrote that it 'remains merely a stepping stone to achieving the ultimate goal of optimising the intimate inter-relationship between structure and function that is required in all systems whether biological or mechanical to work effectively, remain pain free, robust and healthy' – a perfect example of the mechanical, 'replace the broken part' mindset that pervades some parts of medicine.

So what happened? After all that reviewing, in 2019 the government quietly dropped its plans to stop funding fusion for low back pain, I revealed in *The Age*. Orthopaedic surgeon Professor Ian Harris told me the government's reversal showed that 'Doctors and surgeons have too much power, and the government is scared of them and happy to take the path of least resistance'.

And instead of being restricted to the top tier, fusion would receive broad health insurance coverage. Surgeons did get a restriction: no claiming Medicare benefits for spinal fusion for 'chronic low back pain for which a diagnosis has not been made'. This, as Chris Maher told me, was a bit like putting Dracula in charge of the blood bank. To *operate*, a surgeon merely needed to *diagnose*.

Dr Stephen Duckett, a health economist with the Grattan Institute (which receives sponsorship from private health insurers), told me the policy reversal would drive up private health insurance premiums and public hospital bills. 'Always, when the medical profession is acting in its own interest, they dress it up as acting in the patient's interest,' he said. 'What we're seeing here is a triumph of politics over a patient's long-term interests. The overwhelming evidence is that on average spinal fusion does not help people.'

Spinal fusion is a difficult operation. You're surgically damaging a joint and then trying to encourage the body to repair it. In the old days, they used to put fusion patients in full-body casts while the bone regrew. The large pedicle screws used to secure rods and plates to the vertebrae need to be screwed in hard, in an area surrounded by nerves. If the screw goes in on even slightly the wrong angle it can irritate or damage those nerves, or even damage the spinal cord.

Also, the spine is meant to work as a unit, distributing the load across all the discs and vertebrae. Fusion stops that happening by permanently locking together two sections of the spine. This is a really key problem, because even if the spinal fusion works, up to a quarter of patients need surgery to fix the next spinal level within a decade.[8] For them, fusion locks in a repeated cycle of continuing surgery.

'While it might work temporarily, for a few years ... if you fuse that level, I believe in five to ten years the person is just going to have further problems up the spine,' says Associate Professor Sarah Olsen. 'In my opinion – and there would be a lot of people who disagree – I would be very reluctant to do surgery alone for back pain at all.'

Dr Olsen used to perform fusions for low back pain, she tells me. 'I did not think the patients I saw did well. And I thought, unless my back was unstable, I wouldn't have this done myself. And I cannot persuade someone to have a surgery I wouldn't have myself. And If I wouldn't have it myself, why the hell was I doing this operation?'

Each time you open the body up and start mucking around you invite the potential for something new to go wrong.[9] The spine can become less stable; the hardware inserted in the spine might jab delicate nerves, or break off.

Various studies have estimated the failure rate of spinal surgery at between 10 and 40 per cent.[10] The odds get worse every time you go in for a reoperation. Failure is so common medicos have even invented a 'syndrome' for people with multiple back surgeries who are still in chronic back pain: 'failed back surgery syndrome'. The patient must wear the diagnosis of 'failure' – but really, it looks more like it is the medical system that has failed them.

Gavin Davis, a leading neurosurgeon who has performed many spinal operations, notes that some back pain operations do work well. It's just that fusion itself has not been shown to work unless there's spinal instability. Part of the problem is the issue with diagnosing where in the back the pain is coming from – we really can't, he says.

'We have no way of demonstrating with any degree of certainty with any test known to humanity where the pain is coming from. And no one has ever performed a well-designed trial demonstrating the value of spinal fusion for low back pain,' says Davis.

Why do we keep doing them then? 'Because many of the big multinational instrument companies have a vested interest in maintaining spinal fusion. And there are some surgeons, in Australia and internationally, who receive consultancy payments from these companies. And it is in both parties' interest to continue to do those surgeries,' says Davis.

'I don't want to paint all surgeons as bad. Because *most* surgeons do the right thing. There are certain surgeons who are more aggressive and will perform a lumbar fusion on everything. There are others who will try to follow the science as much as possible. But there is very little evidence supporting much of this.'

What should we do, then? Avoid surgery like the plague? I think Dr Ralph Mobbs offers well-balanced advice: spend at least two years trying conservative therapy, then try pain therapy and psychology.

'And if the pain and rehab specialists feel as though they are not winning, then surgery – and underline this – *may* be appropriate. Not *is*. *May* be – in well selected patients, assuming we can identify a specific pain generator.'

After working through dozens of studies and interviewing scientists and surgeons, I was left with Gavin Davis's words hanging in my head: 'There is very little evidence supporting much of this'. Which brought me back to Dad's back. What happened to him? Did he really need surgery?

Dad was dealing with extreme and chronic low back pain and struggling to walk. His GP first sent him to a pain clinic. Generally that's the right move, says Chris Maher. Pain clinics have been shown to work – but you need one that's going to perform high-quality care. Dad did not get that. Instead, he got opioids – OxyContin – stretching, and a biofeedback machine, treatments Maher describes as 'nonsense'.

Probably because he wasn't getting good care, the clinic did not help Dad's back pain. In fact, so concerned was his GP by the high levels of opioids they put Dad on, he pulled him out after just a few days, and sent him off to see a surgeon. Here's where things get complex.

The surgeon told Dad his pain was caused by a herniated disc. The disc's goo had squeezed out into his sciatic nerve. As we've seen, that's a pretty good reason for surgery. But ... was Dad's pain actually caused by his disc pressing on a nerve? Because if it was pressing on the sciatic nerve, he should have had pain running down his buttock and leg, and a fizzing pins-and-needles sensation in his foot. And he did not. No leg pain at all. When doctors raised his legs, the pain was supposed to sharply increase. It didn't. He was meant to feel numb in his legs, due to the nerves being squished. He didn't.

As Dad and I kicked that around, I could could almost hear things ticking over in his head. No leg pain. No weakness. No sciatica. 'And the surgeon told me that I would need another one done in five years. And it's been 15 years and that hasn't happened.' Dad paused, heaved a big sigh like he always does when he's thinking. 'So now I'm starting to wonder ... whether I ever needed the surgery at all.'

I go back to Maher. Back pain with no leg pain is simply not how pain from a bulging disc shows up, says Maher. It's just ... not. Could Dad be remembering things wrong, he asks? But Dad is adamant. 'I had no pain or weakness in leg or buttock and no lack of feeling or pins and needles in extremities of foot – only pain in the lower back,' he tells me. And his memory fits exactly with mine.

Maher's confused. Rachelle Buchbinder, coordinating editor of Cochrane Musculoskeletal, is more critical. 'He didn't have sciatica or foot drop?' she asks me. I shake my head. 'Oh, that's just criminal.' Would Dr Atkinson, the spine surgeon, have operated if he'd seen Dad's scans? He sighs. It was difficult, he says, because for my father the surgery worked – but in most people it probably wouldn't. Without sciatica, or a major symptom like a spinal fracture, Dr Atkinson would not have operated. 'A lot of people have bulging discs, no sciatica, just like him, and get a pathetic result from surgery.'

Surgery as placebo

If Dad's surgery was never needed, why did he get better?

One possible answer to that may be found in one of the more controversial books published by a surgeon in recent years. *Surgery, the Ultimate Placebo* is a small red-and-white book that mounts a devastating attack on surgery – all the more devastating because the author, Professor Ian Harris, is a highly experienced orthopaedic surgeon.[11]

We usually think of placebos as sugar pills – things that look like drugs but really do nothing. But that's a bit of a misconception: if they really did nothing, we wouldn't have the placebo effect. Instead, what a placebo does is make us *feel* like we're being treated, and that changes our perception of how we feel. Why? Because, Harris writes, we're not actually very good at knowing exactly how our bodies are. Our feeling of good or bad health can often be wildly different from the objective medical reality. Placebos change how we *feel* about our bodies – and can often make us feel a lot better about them.

Harris's case is simple: surgery is a very powerful

placebo, and many of the benefits we chalk up to the scalpel are actually driven by the placebo effect. With surgery, you really know something's been done to you – you can see the scar. We venerate surgeons and, as a society, believe medicine is filled with miracles. And surgery has its rituals: heading to the hospital, sitting on the bed surrounded by clothed doctors, going under, waking up. All these signals tell you that *something happened* – and, as you've been told it's a cure, your brain readies itself to feel better. 'As any magician, illusionist or mind-reader will tell you,' Harris writes, 'we humans are pretty easy to fool.' A 2014 review in the *British Medical Journal* collated 53 placebo-surgery trials. In more than half, people who had a placebo surgery improved just as much as those who'd had an actual surgery.

Remember the evidence back in Chapter 1 about spinal cord stimulators probably not working, despite plenty of people saying they get good relief? A spinal cord stimulator is probably an exceptionally powerful placebo – it's expensive, you program it with a computer (and modern society *loves* technology) and often you can *feel* the tingling stimulation as the device works its 'magic'. It's only when you run a clever experiment, turning off the stimulators or scrambling the settings, that you can see it's not the stimulator that is dulling a patient's pain – it's their mind.

If Dad's back surgery didn't really fix the underlying issue, here then is a possible explanation for how and why he got better. He believed himself fixed, and so he was. The more I thought about it, the more the explanation made sense. Dad's spine was surgically repaired. You'd think he might be more fragile, yet over the next ten years he went from immobile to running half marathons – even playing mixed netball, throwing himself at the ball and sprawling on the floor, full of belief in his body.

Harris – who's worked as a back surgeon and done many spinal fusions – suspects most of the benefits, if not all, from spinal fusion surgery are placebo. Something's been done, so you expect to get better. And we know that if you leave it alone, back pain tends to get better on its own anyway. 'Surgery for back pain has the exact effect I would expect it to have if it were a placebo,' he writes.

At the same time as Dad had the operation, he also changed his life – most dramatically by moving from Melbourne to Adelaide and going from a high-stress job to a low-stress one.

Perhaps those changes, combined with the placebo effect from the surgery, were responsible for Dad's improvement? 'It doesn't seem like his improvement was clearly linked to the surgery,' emailed physiotherapist Peter O'Sullivan. 'More that he slowly got his life back post surgery.'

9   The new science of pain

My pain appeared from nowhere and pushed me into bizarre contortions for years. Dad's pain appeared from nowhere and nearly ruined his life. And then, almost as suddenly as it appeared, it vanished for both of us.

'What were the social, stress or contextual factors going on for your dad over this whole time?' O'Sullivan had written to me in his email about Dad's pain. 'Did any of this coincide with his improvement? These are often the things people don't think of.'

Pain, the physiotherapist seemed to be saying, was a lot more complex than we thought. But it wasn't until I took a deep breath and really dived into the world of pain science that I realised how wrong we are about pain – and how much we have to learn.

'17th-century thinking'

In the house I grew up in, a battered ex-housing-trust property in Adelaide's northern suburbs, half done in fake wood inlay and the other half in floral wallpaper, there was a badly renovated bathroom. Some malicious ex-owner had thought to combine a pebbled floor, baby-blue tiles and yellow wallpaper in what amounted to a vicious assault on the senses of anyone who needed a leak. At the door, there was a slight ledge to hold the pebbled floor. It was wooden, and about 10 millimetres high – the exact height, as if designed that way, of a young boy's toe.

I was born lanky and never grew into it, and my mind was always elsewhere. That little ledge became my personal hill to die on, again and again. Each foot has something like 7000 nerve endings, with what feels like a concentration in the big toe. Mine has less than the average now because I keep repeatedly stubbing them out on that damn ledge.

What happened when I kicked my toe?

Everyone knows the answer: nerves register the sensation and shoot it up our spinal cords and into our skulls, where an explosion of pain immediately blossoms in our brains. This idea of pain was popularised by 17th century French philosopher René Descartes, he of 'I think, therefore I am' fame. Descartes, who in engravings wears a flamboyant mop of hair, imagined the pain system as a series of threads, with pain at one end opening a valve inside the brain (he replaced nerve signals with 'animal spirits' … but the original concept was there).[1]

His theory set the course for how society thinks about pain right up until the present day. You can still find it in textbooks today (everyone overlooks the spirits thing now). Unfortunately for him and for us, it's totally wrong. It's not how pain operates at all. This fact has been staring us in the face for a long time.

For decades, scientists have known about phantom limb pain – the experience common to most amputees of vivid pain in their amputated limb. They can even describe it: burning or pinching or twisting or itching, right on the little finger of the arm that does not exist. If the nerves have been severed, how can the phantom arm still itch?

Explain that, René.

Pain scientists moved on from Descartes' way of thinking about pain long ago. But that new way of thinking about pain has yet to trickle down to the woman on the street. 'Society has a way of thinking about back pain which is still stuck in the 1970s,' says Tim Austin from the Australian Pain Society. 'You could even call it 17th-century thinking.'

Maybe that's because the new theory of pain, when you first hear it, sounds crazy. The current scientific evidence shows pain is not presented to the brain by the body, as Descartes thought, but is instead *produced* by the brain as a response to what it thinks is a threat.

Now, that's not to say pain is imaginary. That could not be further from the truth, pain scientists emphasise. *Pain is real*, and we need to start believing people when they say they're in pain. But pain is not a direct signal from body to brain. There is no pain signal. The brain *decides*. To understand, it helps to start with a story.

Paul de Gelder had been in the water for only a few minutes when he felt something smack into his leg. The navy diver was floating in a wetsuit in Sydney Harbour during a counterterrorism training exercise. He did not think too much of it at first. Maybe the dive boat had come too close and bumped him, or a bit of driftwood had hit him. There wasn't any pain. De Gelder glanced down anyway.

He found himself staring straight into the eyes of a massive bull shark. Its lip was curled back, revealing row on row of white teeth. They were wrapped around his leg.

When you're facing immediate death, milliseconds can stretch into hours. In the stillness of that moment, de Gelder reacted instinctively: he tried to jab the shark in its eyeballs. But his arm wouldn't move. Confused, de Gelder glanced over to his shoulder. There was nothing there. The shark had eaten his arm.

The creature pulled him down into the dark water once, twice, shook him like a rag doll. De Gelder thought he would die. And then – perhaps discovering its catch was not a tasty seal – the shark let go. A near-unconscious de Gelder floated to the surface in a pool of his own blood. A crest of water, flicked up by the shark's fin, hit him in the face, shocking him. He realised he wasn't dead – and started fighting for his life.

As his body spun in the water, the lights of the dive boat came into focus. De Gelder started swimming towards it, swimming with one hand, holding his bloodied stump out of the water so the blood did not bring the shark back to him. He kicked hard, but one of his legs didn't seem to be working well either. De Gelder ignored it. He made it back to the boat, somehow, where his crew pulled him out of the water and onto the deck.

The enormous damage the shark had done was immediately clear. It had taken his arm and the hamstring from his leg. Survival was just the beginning. Surgeons would later have no choice but to amputate the entire leg. The pain, when they woke him from surgery, was enormous; he begged his mother for a gun to shoot himself. 'I wished that the shark had killed me,' he would later tell *Men's Health*.

But de Gelder didn't kill himself. He held firm against the pain, and eventually got on top of it, diving head-first into rehab. He's now a campaigner educating people about sharks – not of their dangers, but their value, and why we need to save the 100 million killed each year by commercial fishers.

Let's zoom in to de Gelder's story, right at the moment he first felt pain – some time after realising the shark was eating him. Not at the moment of attack, when he just assumed he'd been bumped by some driftwood. The tissue damage was instant. But he wasn't in pain. The pain only developed *after* he had somehow swum through the water with no arm or leg.

We see this same story repeated again and again in acts of great heroism, where people can push through injuries that should be disablingly painful. When we stub a toe or bang our funny bone, we're in instant pain. But not for some of the most serious injuries. Imagine trying to swim away from a shark in *agonising* pain – it would be even more difficult than it already is.

It was as though something was giving de Gelder the chance to get away from the shark, rather than generating pain.

The old model of pain can't explain this phenomenon we see time and time again. That's why we need a new model of pain. De Gelder's story is not unique. Battlefields have been full of tales of extraordinary heroism in the face of extraordinary injury ever since humans first started the organised practice of killing each other. But it was not until World War II that scientists started taking this phenomenon seriously.

Anaesthetist Henry Beecher was serving in a field medical unit at the Battle of Anzio, an amphibious landing at a fishing village on the western coast of Italy that soon degenerated into a meatgrinder, the Allies trapped on the beach under unrelenting German fire. Beecher's job was to care for the wounded, of which there were many. He often had little to offer them. For one young man, whose mortar-shell wounds looked like a meat-cleaver had been taken to his body, all Beecher had to offer was a low dose of a barbiturate sedative – far too low to dull the pain. Yet the young man settled, science journalist Paul Biegler writes in his examination of chronic pain, *Why Does It Still Hurt?*[2]

Amid the carnage, Beecher managed to put together a study of the badly injured. Three-quarters of men, despite their injuries, said they were in so little pain they didn't need any pain relief. A decade later, now safely home, Beecher redid the study at Massachusetts General Hospital; nearly every patient undergoing surgery asked for painkillers.

That study caught the eye of Patrick Wall, a scientist working just up the road at Massachusetts Institute of Technology, now usually known as MIT. Wall had also been thinking about the power of distraction – how a parent, when confronted with a child crying after a fall, will often try to distract them with a toy. The method works. And then there's the natural reaction to injuring yourself, which is to vigorously *rub* the bruised elbow. It's weird, but it *works,* Wall realised.

Wall and his colleague Ronald Melzack put all these ideas together in perhaps the most influential pain study of the last 100 years, published in *Science* in 1965.[3]

Their theory: our spinal cord – the superhighway ferrying nerve data up to the brain – is not just a passive player in pain. It contains a series of gates; each gate can swing from fully closed to fully open. As they open further, more pain-related information gets sent up to the brain. They called it 'gate control theory'.

Crucially, these gates are all controllable. The best example is touch. 'If you slam your hand in a car door, your immediate reaction is to start rubbing it,' says Professor Brett Graham, a pain researcher at the University of Newcastle. 'The gate control theory suggests what is happening is the touch signals were switching on the gates.'

Touch is primitive compared to the other tools your body has to open and close gates. The brain itself can send signals down into the spinal cord, turning up the intensity of pain. 'Things like stressful situations' cause the brain to send signals to open those gates, says Graham. Or the brain can shut those gates. It simply says 'No, I don't want to hear any signals that sound like pain right now.' Natural opioids and morphines, as well as serotonin, can all be sent down the spinal cord to dull any pain coming back the other way.[4]

This might be what happened to Paul de Gelder. His brain simply decided he couldn't afford to be in pain, because he needed to get the hell away from the shark that was trying to eat him.

Pain scientists now believe 'a lot of the upstream processing is at least as important, maybe more important, than the ... signals that come up from below', Associate Professor Michael Vagg, former dean of the Faculty of Pain Medicine, ANZCA, tells me.

A revolution in pain science

Just about everyone I speak to about pain keeps giving me the same name: Lorimer Moseley.

'He started all this. He's got some sort of cult-like pain rehab program. He's riding around Australia on a pushbike.' Moseley is a scientist with actual fans. At the mention of his name, in the middle of a serious conversation, one pain psychologist actually lets out a small squeal of excitement. 'He is *legit*', she tells me.

And indeed, when I finally got onto Moseley, he was in the middle of a bike trip – through Burnie, a mining and timber port on the northern coast of Tasmania. Behind him, a convoy of pain professionals – also on bikes – and Moseley's 'Brain Bus', a mobile pain-neuroscience lab.

Moseley is one of the world's top pain researchers and now works as a Bradley Distinguished Professor, Professor of Clinical Neuroscience and Chair in Physiotherapy at the University of South Australia. He's authored more than 400 papers, seven books, and dozens of book chapters. His research has won medals and awards on every continent.

He badged his bike trip as a 'Revolution', and that's really how he sees it. In the last 20 years, he says, important discoveries in pain science have revolutionised the entire field. People need to *know* about it. 'The critical, missing link, is giving people an understanding of what modern pain science says,' he tells me. 'And it's so counterintuitive.'

So he decided to get on his bike. Moseley's travelling roadshow, Pain Revolution, pulls in at rural townships and isolated hamlets. They book the local town hall, set up a few metal chairs and trays of sandwiches, and invite the locals down to hear about how pain works.

Pain, says Moseley, is like an alarm system. A danger signal. A way for the brain to whip us into action to prevent something bad happening. Kick a table with your knee and your brain sends you a quick signal to say 'Hey, stop doing that – you're going to damage yourself.' There are no 'pain signals', only 'danger signals'. The brain interprets that danger signal, along with all other information available to it, and *decides* whether to generate pain. This is Moseley's crucial insight.

'It is the brain which decides whether something hurts or not,' Moseley writes in *Explain Pain,* his highly readable book for people with chronic pain. '100 per cent of the time, with NO exceptions.'[5]

Think about hunger, or thirst, or love, says Moseley. Do you think those feelings come from our stomachs or mouths or hearts? Of course not. Our lived experience is generated by our brain.

Try an experiment: press a a fingernail into the sensitive skin on the back of your hand. The pain starts well before you actually penetrate the skin. You can have quite a painful experience without ever drawing blood and without doing any damage. The pain is a *warning* something bad will happen if we don't take action – in this case by not jabbing your thumbnail into your hand.

'The purpose of pain is protection – it's not detection of damage,' says Moseley. 'If it was only about detection of damage, we would die. Pain stops you doing something before the damage.'

Indeed, some people are born with a rare condition meaning they feel no pain. Quite unlike the comic book hero who is impervious to pain, these people need to be much more careful of injuring themselves, because they never realise when they are doing themselves damage.

'Life threatening injuries are usually pain-free,' Moseley says. 'Think about that. I'm talking about a limb being blown off. Until you were safe, you're pain free. And once your life is safe, you experience enormous pain. The brain is smart enough to know that if it creates an experience that makes you look after an arm that's just been blown off, you'll die. And so it doesn't create that experience.'

I think of Paul de Gelder, half-eaten by a shark, but not feeling much pain. His brain, Moseley is saying, simply decided that generating a huge amount of pain right now was not going to help him survive. The same thing happens to soldiers injured on the battlefield: the brain simply says, no, pain would not be useful right now.

The pain scientist Joshua Pate tells me about strange phenomena he sees in his clinic. Like footballers with sore knees – but they only hurt after the game has finished. Or people with back pain who tell him it hurts to bend down toward the toes. But then he'll ask them to bend side to side – and the pain isn't so bad.

'They look at you wide-eyed and say, "Why did that happen?"' says Pate. The answer, he tells them, is the brain is only predicting that pain is a helpful feeling upon a front-bend when standing up. 'You've never done that movement lying on your side, so there's no memory to rely on. And you aren't as likely to feel pain when you're distracted by the excitement of a football match, when your priority is to compete and play. So the movement can be the same, the tissues involved can be the same, but our experiences can be totally different.'

Our brains are getting information from our nerves all the time, and adding that to other data about where we are, what we're thinking, what we're feeling, our memories. The brain's pain system is trying to predict the world based on (a) the data coming in from the nerves and (b) everything else the brain knows about the situation, including its memories of what has happened in similar situations in the past. Pain is the result of our brain's complex processing of all those data points across many regions of the brain involved in touch, movement, emotion, even memory; scientists call this combination the 'pain matrix'.

One of my favourite experiments demonstrating this was run in 1997 at Baylor College in Texas.[6] A team of scientists brought volunteers into a small room filled with ominous-looking medical equipment. The volunteers took a seat facing a big machine with the foreboding label 'SHOCK GENERATOR' on the front. The machine was wired to the volunteers' heads via two large electrodes, electric chair style. But don't worry, the scientists said, they'd be turning the voltage right down – you should only feel a nasty headache. Then the scientists flicked the shock generator on. A low electric hum filled the room. Slowly, the scientists inched the big control knob up and up, all the way to max.

Most of the volunteers later told patients they felt pain from the electrodes, often tingling or pulsing. Some even said they felt pain in other areas of their body. Most reported the pain increasing as the knob was turned. But the machine wasn't real. The electrodes were just wires. No one was shocked. And yet most people in the experiment felt pain. Why? Because their brain was putting all the information together – like the knowledge a big machine was apparently shocking them – and deciding 'I don't want this to get out of hand, time to make some head pain'.

If the brain thinks a part of the body is under threat, it generates pain. If it thinks we're safe, it drops pain levels. This is really key – because it opens a window to treatment. Chugging along at the back of Moseley's motley caravan is the Brain Bus. Moseley's team will invite locals inside, where a series of experiments is designed to show the difference between perception and reality when it comes to pain.

'Your brain constructs everything you feel and see as a best guess – and sometimes it gets it wrong. And you cannot tell the difference,' says Moseley.

One favourite: the shrunken hand. Moseley actually did this as a scientific study. He got ten people with chronic arm and hand pain to do hand exercises while staring at their sore hand. Then he got them to do the same exercises again while peering at their arm through a set of binoculars. Each pair of binoculars had different lenses in them. When the lenses made the image bigger, Moseley's volunteers reported the pain was more severe. When the lenses shrank the arm, the volunteers reported the pain easing off.

A cute psychological trick? Nope. Moseley went back and measured the swelling on the volunteers fingers. Those who had seen bigger images had *more swelling*.

The point, Moseley tells me, is 'the brain knows vision is

a very precise source of information, so it can pay particular attention to it.'

Remember the counterintuitive data suggesting that people with back pain who get scanned can somehow end up in more pain? This phenomenon might explain it. Our brains take the data – a blackened disc, say – and start to amp up any warning signals coming in from our back.

Stiffness represents another intriguing case study for the role of the brain in pain. I find my back stiffens in the days or hours before pain comes on, almost to warn me I'm overdoing it, and then after the pain the stiffness lingers for days or weeks. I always thought of stiffness as the body's reaction to back pain: something hurts, or is damaged, so we're going to lock the spine up for protection; either that, or I'd overloaded a joint in my spine. Some people with the worst stiffness say they can feel their jammed-up joints grind together.

But new evidence suggests the source of stiffness, like pain itself, is rooted deeply in the brain.

In 2017 a team led by Associate Professor Tasha Stanton at the University of South Australia recruited 15 patients with chronic lower back pain and long-term back stiffness and matched them to 15 healthy volunteers. The researchers built a machine they called 'the indentor' – 'It sounds like it should be in a Star Wars movie,' Stanton jokes.[7] A cross-rack holds a pneumatic arm, which pushes down gently, directly on the vertebrae, testing how stiff each spinal joint is.

The conclusion was remarkable: there was no difference between the two groups.[8] The machine's sensors simply could not find any true mechanical stiffness, even in the people who said they felt the stiffest. 'The feeling of stiffness may not actually reflect the state of their back,' says Stanton.

Next, Stanton's team told her volunteers they were going to apply modest pressure to their spines via the machine, and asked them to estimate that pressure level. People with back pain consistently estimated they were feeling more pressure – about 60 per cent more – than they actually were, and were more sensitive to changes in pressure. 'The stiffer the back felt, the more they overestimated force,' says Stanton.

What does all this mean?

First, it means the feeling of a stiff back is driven by the brain, not only the joints. A 'protective perceptual inference', Stanton calls it.

The theory is this, says Stanton: when you have a sore back, there is a perceived need to protect it from things that could potentially injure it. This may include reducing movement of your back in daily life. And what's a great way to reduce movement? Making the back feel stiff.

The feeling of bone grinding on bone we feel, Stanton's experiment suggests, is a real sensation, but is shaped by more things than we might realise. The stiffness is a creation of our brains that can be influenced by information coming from the back but can also be profoundly influenced by all the other sources of information around us. How do we know this? When Stanton's team paired the sound of a creaky door with the pressure applied to the back, people were even more protective of their backs.

'What's going on in the brain can be, sometimes, more important than what's going on in the painful area,' Stanton told an audience in 2017.[9] 'Particularly when it's a chronic condition.

The joints in the spine themselves are not necessarily damaged or worn or gummed up. 'Truly stiff joints, joints that don't move, are usually not painful. You don't feel stiffness in them,' says Moseley. 'Stiffness is just another perceptual inference.'

'I think this has quite compelling implications for how we treat back pain,' Stanton tells me. The experiment suggests that it's not just the back that's making us stiff, but the brain – and therefore, in treating stiffness, we need to consider the brain. If we can edit the information our brain receives – maybe even change the things we believe – we may have a powerful new way of addressing back pain.

Pain is contextual

Pain is generated by the brain taking into account all the data available to it. This means it is *contextual*. Your pain changes depending on what's going on around you. In serious violinists, Moseley has found, fingers on their left hand are more sensitive to painful stimulation than their right hand.[10] Why? Because the left hand is more important than the right to their career – to playing the violin. The brain is more concerned with protecting one hand than the other. Our brains make these calculations all the time. Athletes don't seem to suffer much from minor injuries that allow them to keep playing, but if they 'do their knee', tear an ACL, something that could end their career, you'll often see them burst into tears. In other pain studies, men were shown to have higher pain thresholds if the experiment was being run by a female scientist! Women recovering from breast surgery feel more pain if they think the pain is being caused by their cancer returning than those who don't – regardless of whether the cancer is actually coming back or not.

Or how about this? Moseley's team asked people to squeeze their own fingers to produce pain that was about a 3 out of 10.[11] Then they had a friend squeeze the person's finger with the same level of pressure. The people reported they were in more pain. Then a stranger entered the room and squeezed the finger with the same amount of pressure. The people reported they were in so much more pain – presumably because the brain was suddenly worried about this strange and threatening new person.

The experiments go on, each more mind-bending than the last. In another, Moseley had a series of volunteers sit in a darkened booth, facing two light globes, one blue, the other red. Then he touched an ice-cold bar of metal to the back of the volunteers' hands – ouch! – and asked them to rate the pain on a scale from one to ten.

When the red light was turned on, the volunteers reported feeling dramatically greater amounts of pain, 'up to twice as much as when the light was blue,' Moseley says. When the red light turned on before the bar was introduced – warning the brain something bad was about to happen – the volunteers felt more pain.

'If pain was only about detecting damage, that experiment would not hurt at all, because we don't damage anyone with the rod,' says Moseley. In each experiment, the stimulus was exactly the same, but the feeling, the pain experience, was different. What changed? The information received by the brain. The *context*.

If you start to view pain as a warning sign, something separate and distinct from any signals coming from the nerves – well, your whole view of pain starts to really change. Like, if there's no 'pain signal' … what determines whether a feeling, like having your fingers pushed back or your joints cracked, is painful or pleasurable?

The answer, says Stanton: it's all about context. Think of massage. Massage can be painful. You're paying someone to find all the sore spots on your back and jab them as hard as they can with their elbow. If someone walked up to you in the street and started jabbing you with their elbow, I bet you wouldn't enjoy it. You'd think you were being mugged!

But for some reason we find that particular pain pleasurable. That's because, Stanton says, our brain is getting lots of information about massage – that we know it's good for us, that it's being administered by a trained professional – that suggests this pain is good for us. The same thing goes for scratching an itch. 'It really hurts,' she says. 'But it's a pleasurable experience. Any time anything happens to us, we're putting it into context. We're expecting the pain will happen. If you heard a noise outside, it matters if you ordered pizza. Are you expecting the pizza? If not, oh crap – it's a burglar.'

By now, there is likely a thought – an angry one – racing through your head.

So you're saying my pain isn't real? That it's all in my head?

No. That is not what the science says. The evidence we have is that pain is very, very real. The brain plays a key role. But the pain is still real. 'All pain – the pain of grief, the pain of injury – is psychological. But that doesn't mean it's caused by psychological processes,' says Professor Michael Nicholas, director of pain education at the Pain Management Research Institute.

Why can't we accept this? Why does society constantly demand people show evidence of injury to accept they are in pain? Why is a person with cancer in *real* pain but other people in pain are looked at sceptically?

In the 19th century, doctors generally believed people when they said they had chronic pain – even if they couldn't find a cause.[12] As medicine developed, neurologists started to come up with specific tests for nerve pain. And if they couldn't find a specific cause, well, they didn't want to deal with it. Chronic pain shifted into the realm of psychoanalysts, who were only too happy to diagnose a person in pain with a mental or emotional disease. By the 1920s, doctors had come to think of people with unexplained pain as deluded, mad, drug-addicted or just plain lying.

The 'disease–illness paradigm', as it is known, demands that every problem should have a direct physical cause.[13] If medicine can't explain something, it isn't real. For hundreds of years, society has stigmatised those with chronic pain. There's a use-by date on sympathy. Family, friends and bosses come to doubt whether the pain is real, wonder why we can't just get over it and move on – so much so, the person in pain starts to wonder if they really are mad.

Another part of the problem is political. Governments run disability systems. Imagine the payments they'd have to make if they accepted people's pain experiences. Instead, governments use sceptical doctors who demand evidence of a physical injury or something on a scan. One way a person can qualify for disability support in Australia is if they have evidence of a bulging disc, which flies in the face of evidence that many people *without* back pain – people who have *never* had back pain – have bulging discs. A person's own lived experience of pain 'must not be solely relied on', the guidelines say. This demand is now 'sagging under the immense weight of scientific progress', Moseley has written in a paper with Seamus Barker.[14]

Pain does not mean damage

What does the new theory of pain tell us about back pain?

To start with, I think it's more important for what it tells us back pain is *not*. Pain does not mean there is damage. You can have damage without pain – think of Paul de Gelder getting chewed up by the shark – and you can have pain without damage. This is a really important idea, because it explains why many treatments for back pain that try to target damage – damaged disc, damaged nerve, damaged spine – have been so spectacularly unsuccessful, and it explains why so many people with nothing on the scan can be in prolonged pain.

If we accept this, it changes how we think about preventing and recovering from back pain. To prevent back pain, we need to build strong, resilient minds. We need to look for pain's context: anxiety, stress, fear. And then find ways of treating those issues. If we're going to treat back pain, we need to involve the brain.

10 The mind–body–back connection

Dr John Sarno was called a lot of things over his long career. Guru. Quack. America's most famous back pain doctor. 'Rock star of the back pain world', in CJ Ramin's prose.

Sarno rose to prominence in the 1980s and '90s in America after penning a series of books on back pain, focusing on what he termed the 'mind–body connection'. Sarno was a maverick. Working at a time when everyone was obsessed with the disc, he rejected the dogma of the day and argued that much back pain was driven by psychological and emotional problems. He believed, writes the science journalist Julia Belluz, the 'brain distracts us from experiencing negative emotions by creating pain'. If a feeling was simply too overwhelming to process, or too threatening to acknowledge (Sarno contended that one of the main feelings behind chronic pain was unconscious rage), the brain would distract you from it with pain. Sarno called this 'tension myoneural syndrome', or TMS.

His colleagues were unimpressed. There really wasn't much hard evidence for what Sarno proposed, and he was uninterested in doing the high-quality research needed to prove (or disprove) his theories. 'It made no sense to a lot of scientists and physicians,' Howard Schubiner, head of the mind–body medicine program at Providence Hospital in Michigan, told Belluz.

That didn't stop Sarno. Many thousands of people around the world credit their back pain recovery to him – like many alternative health gurus. Sarno died in 2017. Like many quacks, you'd expect history to quickly forget him.

But here's the thing. A lot of Sarno's ideas are now starting to be proved by modern back pain science. 'The science is catching up to Dr. Sarno,' Schubiner told Belluz. Sarno's 'dos and don't', for example, include such mainstream tenets as 'Don't think of yourself as being injured; and resume physical activity as soon as possible, as it won't hurt you.'

And Sarno's key idea – the linkage of mind and body and back – is at the centre of modern back pain science.

Pain and the brain

We know most back pain isn't caused by a problem with the spine or disc. Where does it come from, then? Likely from a simple injury – a twist, a tweak, a strain, a tiring of the muscle, says Lorimer Moseley. The back is very strong, but we put a lot of load on it during everyday life, and the odds are at some point we'll hurt it – just like I might hurt any muscle I use all the time. Although muscles are hard to injure severely, they have lots of nerves in them. And they're in a fairly sensitive place. 'Biologically, if I was designing a body, and I wanted to make sure the spinal cord was very well protected, I would put a lot of alarm bells around it, and I would make sure if we got any messages to the control centre we would act fast and act hard,' says Lorimer Moseley.

It is at this point, Moseley thinks, paths diverge.

The vast majority of people will endure a couple of weeks of back pain and stiffness. They might miss some work, bend over less, pop a few Panadol. Over time, they will naturally recover. The other group – about a quarter of people who find the pain is so bad they go see their GP – won't recover.[1] They'll get stuck. The answer to why lies not so much in the muscle and bone but in the connection between back and brain. If we're in pain too long, the proper functioning of the pain system, the balanced connections it has with our other systems, can start to break down.

When we're born – even before then, in the womb – our brains are rapidly building new connections between neurons. Encoded in these connections are new knowledge, new memories, new skills. At night, as we slumber, the connections we haven't used much are pruned back. Unused skills grow rusty. Memories fade.

What's all this got to do with pain? Pain is generated by the brain. And the brain is great at adapting and strengthening well-used connections. You can see where we're going. If your brain is regularly telling you your back hurts, over time it will *get better and better* at telling you exactly how much it hurts.

'The longer you have pain, the better your system gets at producing it. Which means that body part gets more and more protected,' says Moseley. 'If we keep running the neurons, the brain cells that produce pain, they get better at producing pain. They become more and more sensitive, so we need less stimulation'

'The pain system is designed as a warning signal. That's what acute pain is,' says Professor Jason Ivanusic, who heads a lab at the University of Melbourne focused on pain.

'There are interactions between the warning signal and many different parts of the nervous system. But even after the problem causing the warning signal resolves, there can be a leftover of the interactions coded somewhere in the nervous system.'

That's part of the reason why people can still be in pain even after their injury has healed, or experience pain in entirely different parts of their body. People with chronic back pain tend to find experiences that have nothing to do with the back – like getting an injection in their shoulder – more painful than people without chronic pain; there's even some evidence people with chronic back pain taste sour things much more intensely. The whole sensory system has been wound right up.

This is not how pain is designed to work. Your pain, which was meant to be a short-term alarm to protect you *now* is now switched on all the time and getting louder. A little bit of pain over a long period of time can become worse and worse until it swallows up your life. 'That's why chronic pain conditions are really hard to treat. You've treated the sore back at the level of the back, there's no visible injury anymore, but you still feel pain. And that's likely because there's still activity happening in your nervous system despite there not being any injury,' says Dr Kelsi Dodds, a pain researcher at Flinders University. But the systems breakdown in chronic pain can be more complete than just an out-of-control pain system flailing away. In some people, the relationship between back and brain breaks down altogether.

In the early 2000s, while much of the back pain field

remained focused on discs and vertebrae, a new breed of back pain researcher was quietly emerging. They were interested not in the spine but in the brain. High-quality brain imaging technology was just starting to be rolled out widely. One key new innovation was functional magnetic resonance imaging, or fMRI, which can essentially watch the brain's actions in real time. The researchers pointed them at the brains of people with chronic back pain – and in an instant those who'd made guru-ish claims about mind–body–back connections had hard evidence. Because the brains of people with back pain looked *wrong*.

A number of studies turned up evidence of reduced grey matter in the brain stem and somatosensory cortex, with a strong correlation between these changes and pain intensity. Changes could be seen in the thalamus, the brain's central hub for movement and sensory data, that look not dissimilar to those in people with Alzheimer's.

All this seemed stunning at first, but with more research scientists have a more balanced perspective. Our brains are highly plastic, changing with our lives; if you're in chronic pain, your brain will change to reflect that. We need to be cautious about overinterpreting brain scans.

That said, there's one part of the brain that has a lot of scientists very excited.

'We see changes in brain areas that are involved in formulating our body image, how the body feels to you. The data is pretty consistent in showing there are changes in how the back is represented at a neuronal level,' says Professor Benedict Wand, coordinator of musculoskeletal studies for the physiotherapy program at the University of Notre Dame Australia.

Other researchers are particularly excited by evidence that a particular part of the brain, the primary somatosensory cortex, might be out of whack in people with back pain. The primary somatosensory cortex is responsible for receiving sensory information, like touch, from around the body; each part of the cortex is mapped to a certain part of the body. In people with chronic back pain, this map is all messed up; the size of the region associated with the back is much larger than it should be, overlapping into other areas that are meant to be linked to the leg. On the map of the body, the brain has lost its place. People with chronic back pain struggle to identify subtle touches and sensations on their back. They also struggle to identify letters traced on their back and struggle to identify how other people are moving their backs. Some even report they feel like their back is no longer a part of their body; for these people, the breakdown is truly complete.

Throughout the day, your brain gets lots of information from nerves across your body. Most of the time, these nerves are simply saying 'Everything's fine down here, boss'. So they get ignored. But imagine if that reassuring normal signal cut out. It's not hard to see how the brain could get worried about the back. Worse, if there's a danger signal but nothing else, the brain is going to end up focusing on that.

'We get into a situation where the back feels really bad to us. That feeds into our cognitive models of a back that's worn out and broken down,' says Professor Wand. 'The information streams that suggest a healthy back are diminished, while information streams that suggest danger are upregulated. That's the view of the science today.'

If the tight connection between back and brain becomes

riddled with static, a few bad things can happen. First, you can lose the sense of exactly where your back is in space. 'That might lead to aberrant movement patterns, which might load the back up abnormally,' says Professor Wand. Without effective feedback going back to the brain you could end up tensing muscles more than you should. 'We're not connected to that area. We are not exactly sure what's going on. Some of the pain is a manifestation between what we planned to happen and what actually happened as we move and load our back.'

Other researchers are exploring a similar connection breakdown in the motor cortex, the part of the brain that guides our movements. When researchers expose animals and people to sharp but non-lasting pain, they see a rapid change in the cortex and the pathways that link it to the injured muscles; the area responsible for moving the injured muscle *shrinks*. This change can happen just 15 minutes after injury.

'The outflow [of information] from the brain decreases. And that might actually change the way you move,' says Dr Rocco Cavaleri, a physiotherapist and neuroscientist who leads the Brain Stimulation and Rehabilitation Lab at Western Sydney University with fellow neuroscientist Dr Simon Summers.

It's possible that in people with chronic back pain this link is never fully repaired. 'The tissue isn't aligning with the brain's response. So now you're generating these abnormal patterns to avoid pain that isn't there,' says Cavaleri.

Why does this happen to some people and not others? It all comes down to that first jolt of back pain, Professor Wand suspects. Some people get a particularly bad shot of acute pain – really nasty stuff, enough to make you think something might be damaged, especially if the pain hangs around for a couple of weeks. If this happens at a time when you're getting told something scary about your back – perhaps a doctor is pointing to a blackened disc on a scan – your brain can link the pain to the idea that your back is seriously damaged.

Some people become so worried by this, perhaps because their brain has already lost its connection to the back, that they start to catastrophise, to hold themselves stiff and stop moving. 'You start to conceptualise the problem as irreversible and the back as highly fragile,' says Professor Wand. 'You get caught up in a cycle in which unhelpful thoughts about the back in pain are reinforced by how the back feels to you and the information you receive from the back.'

At the sparkling modern headquarters of Neuroscience Research Australia in Randwick, James McAuley has spent the past few years poking and prodding back pain sufferers to test out just how much the connection between back and brain has broken down.

McAuley has his volunteers lie down on their front and pull their shirts up, before administering what he calls a 'two-point discrimination test'. It is so strange, yet so telling, it's worth trying on yourself to fully understand. All you need is a friend and a paperclip.

First, fully bend the paperclip out into a straight piece of wire, and then sandwich it back together so the wire's two tips meet. Hand the paperclip to your friend, and close your eyes. Ask your friend to jab you, very, very gently, on a piece of exposed flesh. The back works best, but anywhere will do (except the eye). That first jab should feel like a single point, obviously because it is one. Now, your friend needs to jab you a few more times, and then bend the two tips slightly apart (make sure they don't tell you when they do this). Your job is to work out when the tips have been split into two pins. It's harder than you think.

When I had my girlfriend do it to me, my back was quite sensitive to the pin and I picked the split straight away. The next time, I asked her to try to fool me – time the pokes randomly, make them very gentle, separate the wires by only a fingernail of air. The exercise became much harder. But I still got it right more times than not, even on very small distances, and on repeated goes I quickly became much more accurate.

Patients with chronic pain, McAuley has shown, really struggle with this test.

'If you've had back pain for more than three months, the points can go very far apart and you still say there's one point. Your brain's losing the ability to discriminate between those points,' he says. 'That's about your brain processing the information coming from your back in a different way to everyone else, and in a different way to the rest of the body that makes it less precise and less accurate.' People with chronic back pain, this experiment suggests, process sensation in their back differently.

Dad told me he always felt 'twisted' – as though his spine was wrapping around itself, tied up in a bundle of pained and overstretched muscles, so tight it was close to shattering. But it's not really anatomically possible, is it, to walk around with a twisted spine. The 'twist' was in the brain, not in the back.

'That's really common, that people describe their symptoms in a way that's anatomically impossible,' says McAuley.

The brain has lost track of what the back is doing. The back–brain connection has broken down. This is easier than you might think, because the nerve connection between brain and back is already pretty tenuous. There are very few nerves in the back compared to other parts of the body.

'The entire body, basically from the waist to the ground, talks to the brain using the same number of nerves as one of your fingers does,' says Associate Professor Michael Vagg. 'Pain information created anywhere below the waist gets summarised and condensed and summarised and eventually makes its way up to the brain in a highly condensed form. Because the brain only receives extremely pixelated, non-spatially-resolved information from the back, everything that can hurt in your back tends to feel like everything else.'

Added to this is the problem of the basic wiring of the body. You've got all these nerves that run through your entire structure, but most of them terminate in the spinal cord. The cord then pipes messages to the brain. These nerves all run on electricity, and, just like a bunch of copper cables jammed together, will all interfere with each other – you'll get crosstalk between the wires. Macquarie University back pain expert Mark Hancock calls this 'neural convergence'. 'Most people who have back pain feel it in their butt, or in other different places,' says Hancock. 'You've got nerves coming from all these different areas and they join in the spinal cord – so when it gets to the brain, the brain is guessing where it came from.'

Hancock uses the example of someone who's suffering a

heart attack. You know how a common sign of heart attack is pain in the shoulder or the jaw? This is because the brain is encountering novel nerve information and sort of guesses where it's coming from.

It can quickly become a vicious feedback loop. Your back hurts. You move less, to protect it. Your brain gets out of sync with your back, while getting increasingly worried about moving – so you move even less, and your brain becomes even more out of sync. Eventually you end up like Dad, convinced your spine somehow resembles a Twistie.

'The theory is your body is hypervigilant for threats. Everything has become a threat at that stage,' says McAuley. 'And you get a bit of back pain, and then that feeds into your threat perception. If you have pain, and you're afraid of it, and worried about the future, about not recovering, you tend to do badly.'

Undoing what's gone wrong

How do you rebuild the connection between back and brain? McAuley thinks he has a way.

In 2017 McAuley launched a trial, known as RESOLVE, with a roll call of other Australian back pain luminaries, including Lorimer Moseley, Benedict Wand, Matthew Bagg, Chris Maher and Tasha Stanton. RESOLVE takes everything McAuley's learnt about the brains of people with back pain and tries to … well, tries to undo everything that's gone wrong.

Jess, who we met back in Chapter 4, enrolled as soon as I passed on McAuley's card. She calls me, a few months later, excited. She's ten weeks into the 12-week trial. And it seems like it might be working. 'My lower back pain is down to probably a one or two. Going into the trial, it was probably a three or four,' she says.

Half the participants in RESOLVE are on placebo therapy – if McAuley's treatment can beat a placebo, he'll know it works. Tentatively, I warn Jess: she might be on the placebo arm. 'But I really think I'm getting the therapy,' she says. (She was, Moseley later confirmed.)

Jess was expecting something hands-on when she turned up at the Sydney lab where the trial is running. Massage, maybe, or exercise. It's nothing like that. To her, it's an entirely bizarre way to treat back pain – a world away from injections and opioids and surgery. 'They talk about just what is pain, and how you can rethink your brain to better interpret pain. They did a lot of dispelling of urban myths about pain. Like, there's no such thing as good posture, and it doesn't exist at all, and ergonomics is just fake science,' says Jess.

McAuley's team then move onto images of backs under strain. Golfers pinging balls down the fairway. People lifting heavy loads with their backs. People with back pain find these images incredibly uncomfortable to look at. 'Why do you feel uncomfortable?' McAuley's team ask. 'Remember, *this isn't happening to you*. It's just a picture. There's no physical reason you don't like looking at this image.' It's a bit of an aha moment for a sceptical volunteer: the brain really is playing a role here.

Next, his team has patients simply look at a slideshow of images of people's backs. Each image is rotated clockwise or counterclockwise or upside-down. The exercise is simple: say which way the image is rotated. People with chronic back pain tend to struggle at first, but get much faster as the task goes on.

'That internal rotation activates some of the motor areas of your brain. It primes you for moving your back – activating the same networks. People who don't move their backs much, we can get them to mentally rotate their backs without them knowing about it,' says McAuley.

Only then do they move into actual movement training – but again with a brain-focused twist. All physiotherapy is done in front of a mirror, so people can watch their backs bend and fold normally. Again, it's all about rebuilding the brain–back connection. The focus is on 'just practising being normal'. Vacuuming. How to return to sport. Simple stuff.

Then McAuley's staff get out the sticks. The participants would lie face-down on the floor, Jess says, with 12 numbers drawn across their lower backs, close together. McAuley's team would poke them, gently, and they had to identify which number they were touching, and whether the stick was blunt or sharp. The exercise is designed to help the brain rebuild its connection with the back.

Initially, it was very difficult – Jess found herself almost guessing. 'But you get better. That's the amazing thing. Sometimes I really can't get the difference between sharp and blunt – but after a while I got good at that.'

There's homework too. At night, Jess lies on the carpet of her two-bedroom flat in Sydney's outer north, and her husband writes three-letter words on her back with his fingers. She has to pick the words. That one's hard too, but she also seems to be getting better. 'I certainly feel more capable,' she says, a note of pride in her voice. 'I'm moving a little bit better. And energy-wise – on the weekend I made three meals in a row on Sunday. That's something I wouldn't have been able to do previously.' She sounds happy, excited, like she's finally made a step on a journey after spending years trying to find the right direction. I tell her how happy I am for her, and how proud I am of her for not giving up.

Daniel Dos Santos Costa is another of McAuley's trial participants. The Brazilian DJ and festival promoter, 38, had spent 18 years struggling with a sore back – apparently the result of compressing a disc while lifting and loading heavy music equipment – when he found McAuley's trial.

Costa had seen the disc compression on a scan in his doctor's office, and ever since had struggled with pain. Being told the disc probably wasn't causing him pain, and that the real cause of his pain was likely his own thought patterns, was almost a *relief,* he tells me.

'They explained to me we don't have anything in our bodies that sends information to our brain that's sending pain. And that was the key moment of the process,' he says. 'And I remember, in the first session, I left feeling good. In the second, I was feeling better. By the third, I wasn't feeling pain at all – and since then I haven't felt pain at all. I know now my emotions, my stress – even the food I eat – affect how much pain I feel. The thing that changed everything was changing my perception of pain.'

When the results were finally published in *JAMA* in August 2022, they were strongly encouraging. McAuley's 138 patients started out with pain rated at about six out of ten. They finished with a three out of ten – and they beat the placebo group. About half ended up with no pain at all – a total recovery. They were less disabled and felt healthier and happier with their lives. A year later, they were still in less pain, were less disabled, and their quality of life was much better.

'People were happier, they reported their backs felt better and their quality of life was better,' McAuley says. 'It also looks like these effects were sustained over the long term; twice as many people were completely recovered. Very few treatments for low back pain show long-term benefits, but participants in the trial reported improved quality of life one year later.'

Have you got the cure?

'No,' McAuley says. 'Not yet. But we've moved closer to a cure.' The study validates his ideas and points clearly towards even better treatments which put the brain at the centre of back pain – where it has always belonged.

11 Overcoming fear

At the age of just 21, David Williams was told he was on the fast track to spinal fusion.

Williams spends most of his time in an office these days, working as a psychologist in Brisbane, but his gruff accent and blunt talking style betray his background: 19 years as a cop on the beat. Before that, he was a fast bowler. Fastest in the west, just about. Williams was a member of Dennis Lillee's young fast-bowling platoon at the Western Australian Institute of Sport. He had dreams of staring at an Englishman across the WACA's sun-bleached pitch – until his back started to hurt.

Williams was referred for physiotherapy and eventually cortisone injections. None of it helped. Eventually, a scan revealed a pair of fractures in one of his vertebrae. His young spine, it seemed, hadn't held up to the extreme forces of fast bowling. 'I remember them telling me if the injections don't fix it, we're going to fuse your spine,' Williams tells me. 'And that would have been the worst thing in the world. The amount of people I see with a fusion of the spine. Doctors tell them they'll be back on their feet in eight weeks, and it's just crap.'

Williams decided to avoid the surgery, making another pair of sacrifices instead: he gave up on cricket, and he gave up – he thought – on ever having a pain-free back again. He carried his sore back with him through almost two decades in the police force, took it across the country from Western Australia to Queensland and back. He kept going to physios, kept trying to do the exercises they prescribed. His back kept hurting. But he tolerated the pain and got on with life – an approach he now preaches to his patients as a sports psychologist.

'The way I work with my patients is: you've got pain. *So what*. We need to accept what's happening to us, and get on with life,' he says. 'But what I learned is you have to do something to make your pain go away – not do nothing.'

At the end of his studies to become a sports psychologist, Williams accepted a role interning at the University of Western Australia. Knowing that his back would struggle to make the rough, bumpy trip across the Nullarbor, he went to a doctor and had four shots of cortisone into the aching muscles. Miraculously, the back was OK on the drive. And then, as Williams was driving down a suburban street in Perth, he got rear-ended. His back, held tight for so long, rebelled and spasmed. Williams was in bed for days.

When he could walk, he turned up at the office of the local university's physiotherapist. She didn't do anything different, really – gave him the standard mobilisation treatments and the same exercises to do in the gym. Williams sounds puzzled as he tells the story.

'She just – she seemed to put it to me in a different way. Which gave me confidence. For some reason, I was able to do these exercises, which I'd never done properly. And because I was able to do them – it was a focus on my glutes, not my back.

'She was able to get through to me, to get through the fear factor, to do those exercises. And I can honestly say as I sit here with you right now, my back pain is minimal.'

That, Williams believes, was the key to his recovery. Not the exercises or the treatment, though they helped. It was the sudden change in his head that let him confront the thing really standing between him and getting better: fear. Fear of pain. Fear of reinjury.

'You gotta find the right doctors. If you don't find the right physio or psychologist, you'll never listen to them and never trust them, and it won't work.'

Getting better, Williams says, means you have to beat your fear of pain and hurt and damage. You have to face the fear and move through it. To do that, you need people around you that you trust. It won't work otherwise.

Williams now specialises in helping police officers with PTSD. As a former cop, he knows a bit about what they see every day. With them, he's gruff but sensitive. Unprompted, he tells me he sees a lot of similarities between traumatised cops and people with sore backs. Someone with PTSD is so fearful they're unable to live their normal life. Same for back pain.

'Coppers become hypervigilant. They're looking out for threats. It's exactly the same for back pain. When a physio's trying to get you to do something that you don't want to do – bend – people won't do it, because they fear it. So they don't get better.'

What actually drives the pain?

Pain, as we have seen, is partially contextual. It's generated by the brain in response to data from the tissue mixed with everything else going on at the time: stress, fear, anxiety, unhappiness. Understanding back pain's context is crucial to beating it.

'If you look at what predicts long-term recovery – or long-term disability – it's often the psychological factors that have a stronger predictive ability than the injury itself,' says Curtin University's Dr Rob Schütze, a psychologist working as part of a multidisciplinary back pain treatment team.

Post-traumatic stress disorder. Poor mental health. Substance abuse disorders. Even how much you hate your job. These are all firmly established, Dr Schütze says, as things that increase your risk of developing chronic back pain. To treat back pain, we also need to treat the brain; the two are intertwined, and one problem can't be solved without solving the other.

'A disc herniation is a diagnosis, but that's not necessary what's driving the pain. It could be depression, fear, muscle weakness, something else,' says Professor Paul Hodges.

Consider this study from Britain: it linked poor mental health at the age of 22 or 23 with a doubling of the risk of having chronic back pain at the age of 32 or 33. This link even started emerging as early as age 16. The worse your 'malaise' – the number of psychological symptoms you report – the higher your chances of developing back pain. People in that study with a lot of psychological distress at 23 had more than a one in four chance of developing lower back pain a decade later. Those are worse odds than playing Russian roulette.

Mark Hancock estimates that in people with chronic back pain, the physical makes up perhaps 20 per cent of the pain – leaving *80 per cent* to come from the mental component. 'People misunderstand it when we say the brain's involved. We're not saying people are making this up,' Hancock says. 'This is a real experience for people.'

To deal with the mental side of back pain, we first need to *accept* that a mental side exists.

We accept physical illnesses, like high blood pressure, because we can see them as numbers on a pressure cuff. We sign the cast of our colleague with a broken arm. We donate to cancer charities. But we're only now starting to take people's mental health seriously – rather than just expecting them to cheer up.

Part of this comes from the dominance doctors and surgeons have enjoyed in our society. The modern medical approach is: find the underlying problem and treat it, either with scalpel or pill. But if an illness is partially or wholly influenced by the brain, these treatments won't work well, or at all. This can leave a doctor or surgeon in a bind. They can't fix the problem. It's all too easy to simply blame the patient; the pain was never real, or they never wanted to get better. Society, led by this dominant medical view, has followed along. If a doctor can't find a problem, well, *you must be faking.*

Society has taken great strides in accepting mental illness in the last few years. But we're yet to fully accept the role that our brains can play in pain and disease.

When I start to tell people with chronic back pain about the incredible new scientific links being discovered between that pain and the brain, they often get angry or upset. Dad certainly did. 'So you're saying it's not real? That it's all in my head? Well, let me tell you buddy ...' They don't feel believed.

'If there's a psychological component, the implication in our society is it's not real,' says Professor Michael Nicholas of the Pain Management Research Institute.

Australia's government-subsidised medical system doesn't help. People are only entitled to a handful of subsidised visits to a dietitian, physio or psychologist a year, but have unlimited access to GPs. 'The message it gives patients is [that] non-drug treatments are not valued,' says Nicholas. 'If you want a real treatment, it has to come from a doctor.'

Another pain psychologist tells me she regularly sees back pain patients who tell her that no one, not even their doctors, will believe them. The pain can't be seen on a scan, so they must be making it up. 'It's really invalidating,' she says.

The effect of this stigma is enormous. 'They're conscious of becoming a burden and stigmatised – always complaining, never getting better,' says Nicholas.

But more importantly, it can prevent people getting better, he says. Because it stops us accepting that our brains play a key role in our pain – and that to treat the pain, we have to treat the brain.

The way you think can put you at risk

The first step to steeling your brain against pain is under-standing the thought patterns that can get you into trouble.

Certain ways of thinking about the world seem to put you more at risk of back pain, in particular something Schütze calls 'low self-directedness'. 'It's like not having a lot of confidence. You feel like things happen to you, you don't make them happen. Your happiness is dependent on stuff that happens to you, rather than stuff you make happen.' These people tend to blame others for their own problems and are emotionally fragile. Recent studies suggest low self-directedness, and another trait called harm avoidance, could be the two personality traits most strongly linked to the development of chronic pain.

Harm avoidance is exactly what it sounds like. Being constantly worried and fearful, sensitive to punishment and criticism, generally pessimistic. Remarkably, this pair of traits – scared of pain, lacking direction in life – shows up in people who develop different types of chronic pain such as fibromyalgia, chronic tension headache and migraine, and people with nerve pain.

It makes a certain sense that people who are especially fearful of pain end up more likely to suffer from it. To a fearful person, even a small, tolerable amount of back pain must feel like a serious problem, and if it isn't fixed soon it's going to get worse and worse and soon they won't be able to walk. They're worrying about that, and at the same time their pain system is dialling the pain up and up …

All that fear warps us. We become afraid to move and

bend. This just makes the problem worse, as our joints gum up and underused muscles atrophy, while other muscles held tense for too long break down and spasm.

Some researchers are directly attacking the problem of fear. Paul Marshall, the exercise scientist from Western Sydney University, is taking perhaps the most blunt approach: recruiting people with back pain into a power-lifting study. 'We thought, if we're trying to address fear, we should give a program that's absolutely terrifying,' he tells me. 'We've had people [go from] being afraid to lift a towel off the ground to lifting 100 kilograms over eight weeks.'

Marshall had volunteers with back pain work through an eight-week powerlifting program, involving squats, deadlifts and rows – big exercises that I often find scary when serious weight's stacked on. Everyone in his study significantly improved their back pain and disability level – but so did another group who were doing bodyweight exercise. Powerlifting, sadly, does not appear to be a cure-all for chronic low back pain.

However, there are two key takeaways I find interesting. First, you can do powerlifting safely – under supervision – if you have back pain. Second, Marshall's team found that as the volunteers' measures of fear and self-efficacy – similar to self-directedness – improved, that strongly predicted an improvement in their pain. For some people, lifting heavy weights might be what it takes to rid them of their fears.

Beating fear

For some people, beating fear is at the core of their back pain recovery.

When I started talking about my book with Viv, a friend of a friend, I was expecting a glazed look; for young, healthy people who haven't encountered back pain, the idea can seem remote and improbable. But Viv's eyes widened straight away. He'd been struggling with terrible back pain, he told me – until recently, when he'd faced his fear, and changed his life.

Viv's back had never really given him any trouble until one night, after getting 'pretty loose' at a music festival, he awoke stiff, he tells me. At first he didn't think much of it, figured it would pass. 'I'd hurt myself before. I was like "Whatever. You just roll through the pain",' he tells me. He went and played a weekend game of football as normal.

But the pain didn't pass. 'It slowly got worse,' he says, until it was shooting jolts of pain right up his back. And, bit by bit, it started to change his life. He dropped sport. He spent more time lying in bed with a hot pack to ease the throbbing pain. 'I vividly remember driving my car to work and it was just absolutely smashing me,' he says. 'I was just crying in the car going to work, and I was like "Why the *fuck* isn't this getting better?"'

Here's where the fear comes in. Viv told me that more and more he was starting to feel *overwhelmed* by his pain. It wasn't getting better. What if it *never* got better? What if he was *stuck* like this for life?

'The advice I was getting was rest it, be careful. Any time I said anything to anyone it was like "Really, you're too young for that to happen. That's really bad." And that was really triggering to me. I thought I was going to be one of those people. I was pretty scared – I really struggled to sleep.'

At the same time, Viv was working in a stressful job as

a legal aid lawyer. Many of his clients had chronic diseases – including back pain. One client, he recalls, had such a spasm he collapsed in front of him. Stress, pain, fear that you'll be disabled for life – Viv's brain was overwhelmed with bad news and fearful images.

But Viv turned it around by conquering his fear. His first step was a copy of Lorimer Moseley's *Explain Pain,* handed to him by a physiotherapist. He read it with wonder. It helped him understand how the pain system could go so wrong; how he could be in pain without any obvious physical cause. But it didn't make him better. Not at first. For that, Viv turned to a smartphone app called *Curable.* Developed by a team of American neuroscientists and psychologists, the app teaches modern pain science and is focused on understanding pain and reducing the fear and anxiety that go alongside it.

The app included brain retraining and guided meditation, which Viv dived into. There were breathing exercises to stay calm. A self-talk exercise: 'Saying out loud you're safe, you're strong, you're going to get through this, your back can withstand this,' says Viv. And it recommended a name change. 'Pain' had become such a loaded, fearful word. Viv opted, he tells me with a laugh, for 'banana'.

'And so any time it was happening I'd think "A bit of banana there",' he says. It sounds ridiculous. But it was working for him. 'It was taking the fuel away from this trigger word, "pain".'

Recovery took time – about nine months of working on his mind and slowly increasing his exercise levels with a physio before he could really say he was feeling better. But slowly the fear fell away, and so did the pain. Viv is now back doing what he loves: surfing, playing sport, living a rich life. I ask him if he has any advice for people with back pain. Stay calm, he tells me, because you do get better. And remember, the fact the brain plays a key role is a good thing, 'because our brains are easy to change'.

Can pain change the brain?

Some thought patterns can put us more at risk of back pain. But in some people, the reverse seems to happen: back pain causes their personality to change. And that change 'locks in' the back pain.

'A lot of people come to me and say: my family and friends say the reason why I've developed pain is because of my personality, or it lies in myself. And that's a stigma. And it's not true,' Professor Sylvia Gustin tells me.

Professor Gustin, director of the Centre for Pain IMPACT, works on brain scans of people with chronic back pain. Using an MRI machine, she's built highly detailed maps of their brains, and compared them to the brains of people without pain.

The shapes of the grey matter of the two groups had subtle differences in a region called the thalamus. These differences might be enough to amplify pain signals. And they might be enough to change who a person is.

The thalamus lies in the middle of the brain, where it's responsible for putting together all the data coming from your body – eyes, ears, nose, touch, pain – and sending it to the higher parts of the brain, where your consciousness is thought to lie. It also has a regulatory role, controlling how much data gets through. Think of it as a valve.

People with chronic pain have a smaller thalamus, with lower levels of the neurotransmitters that keep that valve tight, Gustin has shown. Their valves are leaky. More signal gets through from body to mind. You can imagine what that means for someone with pain: more pain signals get through. This might explain why chronic back pain can be so awful and debilitating, and why it often seems much worse than the injury itself would explain.

'We call it a loss of inhibition,' Gustin says. 'Every signal from the periphery gets amplified, and results in the ongoing experience of chronic pain.' What's causing the changes to the brain is harder to say. It could be that having back pain causes your brain to change, but Professor Gustin does not believe that. 'My hypothesis,' she tells me, 'is stress.'

When you hurt your back, you get a big surge of stress, Gustin says. I think of my back aching at moments of peak stress, and my dad losing his grip at work. Stress causes the body to release the hormone cortisol, which has been shown in studies to be toxic for brain cells if it stays at high levels in the brain for too long. Essentially, stress reshapes your brain to make you more vulnerable to chronic pain, Gustin thinks. Those brain changes can actually change your personality, making you more fearful and less confident.

The time Dad's back pain was worst overlaps perfectly with when he was at his most stressed. Finished with covering slaughters across Europe as a foreign correspondent for the ABC, he became part of the leadership team at ABC local radio in Melbourne, a government broadcaster always under intense scrutiny from outside, and always seeming to be dealing with budget cuts from within. Then he launched an internal program to cover Australia's many natural disasters – fires, floods, cyclones, earthquakes – which constantly put him in conflict with other powerful departments at the broadcaster. He couldn't get enough time off, and when he did have a holiday, a disaster always seemed to strike somewhere, and he was back in the office. Dad's back was a powder keg waiting to blow.

'You often see back pain begins at a time of someone's life when they're really stressed. They're not sleeping well. They do something minor, they get pain, they get scanned, and the whole thing escalates from there,' says Curtin University back pain guru Dr Peter O'Sullivan.

Stress and back pain

Disliking your job, or finding it mentally or emotionally stressful, dramatically increases your chances of suffering from back pain, evidence suggests. Workplace stress, or feeling like you don't have control over your work, just makes it worse. In 2010, two American doctors, Roger Chau and Paul Shekelle, published a remarkable paper in *JAMA* – a meta-review that pulled together data from 10 842 patients across 20 different studies of lower back pain, looking for the red flags that separate those who would recover from those who would go on to develop chronic back pain.[1]

They looked at everything. Gender. Education. Weight. Whether a person smoked, or had received workers compensation, or even if they worked a particularly physical job. The one demographic variable that best predicted who'd recover and who wouldn't? *Job satisfaction*.

'The evidence is the strongest contributors to persistent pain are in the psychosocial domain – beyond the local physical pathology,' says Tim Mitchell. Mitchell started out as a back pain researcher. Now he leads a staff putting evidence into action at his physiotherapy clinic, Pain Options.

Back when Mitchell worked at a university, he led a study of 170 student nurses, trying to work out who was most likely to go on to develop back pain. Nurses are notoriously prone to back pain: constant movement, limited sitting, large and difficult loads to move all make for a lot of load on the back muscles.

But not all nurses get back pain. Mitchell's team wanted to know why. Posture? Back muscle strength? Core stability? General physical fitness?

The team carefully observed the student nurses, measured the curves of their spine as they sat and stood, looked at how they lifted patients. But here they found little difference between those suffering back pain and those who reported they were fine. They all had similar postures, their backs were all about the same strength, and they were all at the same level of fitness.

What really differed was not the physical, but the mental: stress. People with higher levels of stress were more likely to report bad back pain.

Stress is a normal and important part of our lives. It primes our body for action when we need it, sending adrenaline through our veins. But it's meant to be temporary. If we stay stressed too long, or get stressed too often, we can face a cascade of health problems.

Stress does not always play a role in back pain, says Mitchell. But for some patients, it's a major cause of either the back pain starting, or not going away.

There's a strong link between our neural system and our immune system. Repeated stress can push our immune system into overdrive, which can cause chronic inflammation of the tissues.[2] When someone is struggling with chronic stress, their body often loses its ability to regulate the inflammatory system, evidence suggests.[3]

Stress triggers adrenaline, which can increase muscle tension – bad for people with backs that are already tense. A tense muscle constricts blood flow, starving it of oxygen. In response to a lack of oxygen, muscle cells release bradykinin, a protein that promotes inflammation and ups the sensitivity of surrounding nerves. Stress literally causes pain.

'You can have a brickie that does the same job, day after day, and then suddenly at the end of one day, his back's really sore. If there's no change in physical volume or load to explain the symptoms, we used to think the disc must have given out, something structural happened,' says Mitchell. 'But put a different lens on it: the bricklayer might be lacking sleep, has been generally unwell, their stress levels are high. And that can pre-sensitise your system.'

We know stress can trigger inflammation; some people also hold their stress in their muscles, tensing them up. The back ends up inflamed and tight; bend over one day and *bam*, a muscle spasm. In other cases, people with back pain can get so stressed about it the stress gets in the way of their system recovering.

'They may have really overloaded their back, or [have] a disc protrusion directly compressing a nerve. But their heightened level of distress, including with increased inflammation in the system, delays recovery, doesn't allow the system to calm down again,' says Mitchell.

All this rang true for me. In the most stressed times of my life, my back and neck have reliably ached, with a tension that can't be stretched out. When I was trying to run a university magazine, consumed by looming deadlines, my back rebelled, and I found myself spending long hours on the floor, riding out the spasms.

The prescription

If stress is the trigger for the changes in the brain Professor Gustin sees on her scans, then there's a simple prescription to help treat chronic back pain: stress less.

'Particularly in the acute stage of pain, we need to calm ourselves. We need to work on ourselves that we are not focused 24 hours a day on the acute pain,' she says. She advises practising mindfulness meditation, to learn to separate the conscious mind from the sensations of the body. Think of yourself as the diver, she says, looking down on the blue pool of all your feelings. You have a choice of whether to dive in, or just observe the cool blue surface.

This is, of course, very difficult advice for someone who thinks they've just blown a disc or fractured a vertebra to implement. But remember: the odds are you haven't. Nearly all painful back injuries are just muscle strains that will heal in a few days or weeks. Even the bigger injuries, like a disc herniation, can and do heal by themselves. So hang onto that knowledge and try to relax: that gives your brain the best chance of avoiding stress-related changes.

And if you're dealing with long-term back pain that just won't go away, consider a radical prescription: job change. Is it possible your job is making you stressed and sore and, ultimately, sick? Would you be happier, fitter and healthier doing something else? Soon after his operation, Dad moved us to a less stressful life in Adelaide, with a shorter commute. We have family there. Dad was hoping they could look after him, 'and help Mum if I couldn't walk anymore'. Could that have been as important to his recovery as the operation itself?

Pain and the immune system

If we're in pain for too long, our brains and nerves change in unhelpful ways. But increasingly there's an appreciation among scientists that the problem is broader than just nerves. 'We've always known, since the 1950s, the nervous system changes when you have chronic pain,' says Tim Austin, chair of the Australian Physiotherapy Association's National Pain Group. 'We've worked out in the last decade or so that increasingly it's the *immune system* that regulates the nervous system.'

Scattered across your neural system are a subset of cells called glia – from the Greek word for glue. For a long time, science ignored them. They seemed to do little more than support neurons, and neurons – with their little zaps of electricity – were much more sexy and interesting to scientists. Research in the last 20 years shows this is likely wrong. Glial cells are intimately involved in the nervous system. They support and nourish neurons. They protect nerves from infection. They prune back unused neural pathways. And they are especially involved in pain signalling.

One core insight that unlocked this new area of science:

how crummy we feel when we have a cold or flu. Think about it. Why would having a cold make you ache all over? Why would it make you more sensitive to pain or cold? 'Based on fundamental neuroscience, your brain shouldn't know what your immune system is doing. But we *know* that we feel different,' says Professor Mark Hutchinson, director of the Centre of Excellence for Nanoscale BioPhotonics in Adelaide. (The centre's futuristic name refers to a technique of using photons of light to measure biological processes; Hutchinson is working to build a light-based blood test for pain.)

In Chapter 6, we saw how the nerves that spread through our body send signals back to the spinal cord, which transmits them up to the brain. But we also saw the spinal cord was able to regulate and influence those signals, turning them down or up – like a dimmer on a light switch. It turns out glial cells are central to this process. Almost at every single junction between the nerves that carry signals from your flesh to your brain, immune cells play a 'critical role', says Hutchinson. They can turn those signals up or down; they're so powerful that they can create the signal all by themselves, no flesh needed, he says. 'And this is where chronic pain comes into play.'

When a nerve is damaged, the glial cells become inflamed. The cells can change shape, release pro-inflammatory factors, and lose the ability to do their important nerve-regulation jobs. But unlike tissue inflammation, which can quickly clear, glial cells can remain inflamed weeks and months after an injury. This inflammation can be seen in the nerves of the tissue, the spinal cord, even the brain. 'You have an ongoing stimulus, like inflammation, and that actually causes molecular changes in the sensory nerves. Those molecular changes make the nerves more sensitive to painful stimuli – or they might actually start to detect stimuli that isn't painful and detect that as pain,' says Dr Kelsi Dodds. 'There are these funky things going on with the cells that is changing their sensitivity. The brain starts to see these abnormal signals as painful.' This new biology also hints at why painkillers like opioids, and surgery that targets nerves, often don't work very well for chronic pain: they target neurons, when the real problem may be in the glial cells.

Glia, and the role of the immune system in pain in general, explain another key mystery about pain: why it's so individual. Our lived experiences, even from childhood, can leave indelible marks on our immune system, sensitising it to pain. There's emerging evidence that early life traumas can directly affect the glial cells in the still-forming nervous system, putting them on high alert for the rest of a person's life. Painful procedures in infants – who, insanely, were long considered not to feel pain at all – have been shown to change the way their nervous systems process pain deep into adulthood. Children who experience a lot of stress early in their life have a lower pain threshold as adults, evidence suggests. 'We've always said, in the pain world, no two patients are exactly the same,' says Associate Professor Michael Vagg. 'That's true to a level we couldn't have possibly imagined 20 years ago.'

All this sounds miserable: yet another reason for pain. But within these discoveries, optimism blooms. Because it offers us yet another target in treating chronic back pain: the immune system. And once again, finding ways to destress is the key.

'Globally, we're dealing with a turned-on life. We're working our bodies to an extreme where we only really exercise the on-systems. We hardly ever exercise the off. From an immune perspective, we're operating on the edge of a reactive immune system,' says Hutchinson.

We don't sleep enough. We live stressful lives. We eat unhealthy foods. We don't take enough time to meditate. 'Every single one of the things we enjoy about western life are hits to our physiology. That takes us closer and closer to a load that's more likely to develop a chronic pain state.' Hutchinson's guidance is simple: sleep better. Eat better. He advocates the 5-2 diet, which asks you to fast for two days a week, keeping calories below 600.

'There's now really good evidence coming out around practices such as the 5-2 diet. The immunology is not suppressed – it's balancing.' He also recommends mindfulness, yoga and meditation. 'The Eastern medicines have this right,' he says. 'There's beautiful data out there now showing those types of mindful practices do actually lead to that balanced [immune] response.'

Can pain be inherited or learned?

As the link between the brain, mental health, and back pain became clearer in my research, I became … well, a little more worried about my back. What was spending all day, every day, thinking about back pain doing to my own mindset? Was I likely to become more gloomy, more obsessed, I wondered. Or would my mind end up steeled against pain?

And, I wondered, if you were a young person growing

up in a family where a parent had serious chronic back pain – what would that do to you? I had a neat natural experiment: myself. I grew up with a father trapped in his own dark spiral of back pain. And then I fell into my own dark spiral. Could the two be related?

'What you're saying, we hear quite often,' says Dr Amabile Dario, a researcher at the University of Sydney. Clinicians often see a patient with back pain, she says, and it soon turns out it runs in the family: grandparents, parents, children. Indeed, there's reasonable evidence now showing that a child with a parent struggling with back pain is more likely to develop their own pain – the odds are about 58 per cent, per one study published in *Pain* and led by Dario.[4] Two parents, and the risk is even higher.

The obvious culprit is genes. 'We know they play a role,' says Dario. Sadly, there's not much you can do about that. But there's also some suggestion the parenting environment may play a role too. A meta-review published in *Pain* in 2020 found moderate associations between a parent's protective and 'catastrophising' behaviour, as well as general anxiety and depression, and higher levels of disability reported by their children. Catastrophising here means a parent who simply is unable to cope with their child being in pain; they feel overwhelmed, unable to stand it, worried the pain is a sign something seriously bad is wrong, and yet feel unable to help. As a new parent, I can entirely understand how you can feel that way, watching someone you love suffer. But the evidence suggests it just isn't that helpful.

The science is far from conclusive, and more work needs to be done, but it's interesting, and it fits my life story. Is it possible my father's fears over the state of his back caused me to grow anxious and stressed about mine? When Dad was struggling to get out of bed, was that telling me my back was weak and prone to fail at any time? When Dad was thinking he was about to lose the ability to walk, was that telling me I should be worried any minor twinge might be a sign of long-term damage?

'Kids, they learn by observing. If they're observing their parents talking about pain quite often, being negative about pain quite often, I believe they're likely to do exactly the same,' says Dario. 'Pain becomes something very important in their lives, because that's what they observe in their families all the time.'

What can parents do if they're worried their children may pick up unhelpful messages about pain? Start pushing positive ones, like the power of staying active when in pain, working through the hurt, says Dario. Parents probably can't change a child's pain, but they can help change their lifestyle.

How our thinking affects our healing

Our mental health does not just expose us to a risk of developing back pain. It can also have radical effects on the way we respond to back pain and recover from it – or don't. 'The research is pretty clear now: there's a helpful way to respond to pain, and a not-so-helpful way,' says Schütze, the back pain psychologist. 'The unhelpful way is to freak out. We call it "pain catastrophising". Lots of worry and anxiety, rumination, but also avoidance behaviour. What backs love is to move. If you stop moving, or don't give the backs movement they like, that's when the problems really kick in.'

Everyone with serious or long-lasting pain gets bad thoughts. That's normal. The difference between people who do well and those who don't is the ability to catch those bad thoughts and snuff them out before they lodge too deeply in the brain. They refuse to live in fear. And fear is powerfully dangerous.

'It's when we dwell on them that we get into trouble,' Schütze says. Ruminate obsessively on the bad thoughts and they'll start to become dogma and start informing your whole life. Your life will start to warp around the pain. 'The trick is not to get stuck in that sort of thinking,' he says.

Schütze pointed me to a study he led in 2017 interviewing 15 people with chronic back pain (most of them for at least nine years) and classic signs of pain catastrophising.

Their words are deeply troubling – especially if you recognise your own thoughts in them.

> I spend so much time thinking about it and then, on top of that, thinking that I shouldn't be thinking about it. Then on top of that, thinking I shouldn't be beating myself up about thinking about it. It just gets ridiculous.
>
> – Carly

> If you think the worst and it doesn't get there, that's a positive. But if you're constantly thinking positive thoughts then anything bad happens, then you're not ready, you're not prepared for that. So I prepare myself for the worst, I guess. It sounds horrible.
>
> – Gail

People who struggle with back pain often believe they've lost control of their body and health. Here, Schütze says, is where we need to pull ourselves up. 'We have to encourage people to take control of their own health. If you don't believe you can have much of an influence on your problem, you're not going to try to fix it.'

Leaving your care solely in the hands of your doctor is not the best way to get better. 'Slavishly following that model leads us into trouble,' says Schütze. 'And I think that's why we're in such trouble as a society. Because people are waiting for the experts to fix their problem. We need to empower people. We need to take the focus away from guru-like health professionals.'

Take your care into your own hands, says Schütze. Start with the knowledge that it is extremely unlikely you've seriously damaged your back. Then work on your fear. In the words of Franklin D Roosevelt: 'You have nothing to fear but fear itself.'

How can we remain brave in the face of pain? How can we conquer our fears?

There isn't a lot of direct research on this problem yet. But we can find hints of an answer, I suspect, in a large long-term Scottish study looking at people with high levels of pain. Most of these people, about two-thirds, said they really struggled to live their lives, as you'd expect. But the other third did not. They were in pain but they were still living happy, full lives.

When the researchers went back to these people ten years later, they found they were 25 per cent less likely to have died, even after controlling for things like age and illness. Something seemed to protect them. They were *resilient*.

Other studies offer tantalising hints at how you might access that resilience.[5] Optimism is key – holding an optimistic attitude to pain, no matter how bad. Staying positive. Having a strong purpose in life and working towards it, whether that's career or sport or caring for your kids or being a good partner. Accepting some level of pain as something you cannot change – but that won't deter you from living a good life. Active coping: putting in place strategies to deal with the pain, rather than being controlled *by* the pain.

'It all sounds a bit fluffy, a bit mind-over-matter. But it's got good science behind it,' says Schütze.

People who handle pain well tend to substitute obsessively worrying about the pain with problem solving. They design a plan to fix their problem, and then get to work. That could be a graduated exercise program, or diet changes, or researching how pain works, or enrolling in a back pain class, or finding a good pain psychologist. But it also seems – and this is crucial – that just *having a plan* and putting it into action works. The strategy itself doesn't necessarily have to succeed. Simply by taking action, you start to break the cycle of dark thoughts that go with chronic back pain.

'You come up with a plan and then you do something,' says Schütze. 'It transforms thinking into doing.'

The overarching theme that underpins resilience, says Schütze, is optimism. An optimistic attitude to back pain gives you a buffer against getting stuck in a cycle of dark thoughts – which can make the pain worse – and gives you a push towards taking your health into your own hands, and starting to solve your problems. '"I'll get through this" is much better than thinking "I've slipped a disc and I'm two steps from a wheelchair",' he says.

Chronic pain can generate a negative spiral of pain and fear and depression and anxiety, until you end up at the bottom of a deep well. But a spiral can go both ways. A positive attitude, anchored on the belief you can change your own pain, leads you to doing things – exercise, seeing friends – that are themselves positive and give you a sense of accomplishment. In turn, these generate good feelings, which make you want to do them more, while encouraging the brain to dampen down its pain signals.

'It's easy to withdraw because you're sore, can't do group activities in the same way as before, or you start to feel disconnected from people and insecure,' says Schütze. 'But social support is one of the most protective forces against pain-related disability. We're social creatures. Connection is vital for health.'

12 A different approach to back pain

As we've seen, a lot of back pain medicine does not work. Some might even make you worse. Avoiding it is the first step.

But doing nothing is not enough. What might a modern approach to chronic back pain treatment look like?

After speaking to dozens of experts and reading hundreds of studies, I came again and again to the same two pillars: strong mind, strong body.

The first section of this chapter will focus on acute pain. What to do when you've hurt your back when the pain is at its most intense. These therapies – ibuprofen, heat – may work best in combination as an enabler for the real treatment: exercise. Then we'll look at why exercise and movement is so important to recovering from pain and then building a base to make sure you don't experience it again. We'll look at when a good psychologist can be a valuable pillar of recovery. And finally we'll touch on a couple of the most exciting treatments coming around the corner.

What to do for acute back pain
Apply heat pads and ibuprofen

When I visit Chris Maher in his office in Sydney, he's playing with a pair of what look like incontinence pads. Maher, a deeply serious scientist, flaps them about. I try not to laugh. They are heat pads, he tells me. Simple, cheap; you can buy them from any chemist. 'We just stick them on.'

What's Maher, doyen of the evidence, doing messing around with cheap pharmacy heat pads? He shrugs. The evidence actually suggests they probably help. Cochrane found moderate-quality evidence that heat therapy cuts both pain and disability for people with sharp back pain in the short-term. Allowing the heat to warm up the muscles and joints and then doing some light exercise seems to work even better. The evidence isn't fantastic, but crucially heat – as long as it's not so hot it burns you – comes with very few risks.

Why does it help? I ask Maher. 'I don't know. It feels warm and comforting. And they can get up and move while it's on there. Heat does relieve pain, and we think for back pain, becoming more active does help the process. So this is a combination of the two.'

I used to spend hours lying on my stomach, microwave-hot wheat bag on my back. It was comforting, but thinking back on it, it never really seemed to improve the problem long-term. When the heat wore off, my back would be as sore as ever.

But heat pack technology has come a long way. Maher likes FlexEze heat wraps, lightweight air-activated wraps that stick to the skin and are so thin you can't even see them under a shirt. You could wear one all day, allowing the heat to soften tight muscles. Unlike the wheat bag, you can get up and go with one on.

Combine these with ibuprofen – which, as we saw in Chapter 7, probably helps a little with back pain – and you have a useful treatment for acute pain. Heat and ibuprofen are not cures. They won't fix your back long term. But that's not the goal. Strap on a heat pack, pop some pills, and you'll feel a bit better for a few hours. And then you can use that time to get up out of bed and do something that really does seem like a cure for low back pain: exercise.

Exercise is vital

Compared to everything else we're sold to make us healthier and our backs less painful – surgery and drugs, vitamins and superfoods – exercise is extraordinarily good for us. It works, both as a back pain therapy and as a general way to improve our health.

To understand why, we need to go back. Way, waaay back. Back to the beginning: the dawn of humankind. That's where we'll find the answers to a very strange human paradox: our need to move. If you take the Charles Darwin view of things, exercise makes no sense. Humans, like all animals, are here to take in enough energy to reproduce. Exercise uses energy, and evolution typically goes to enormous lengths to conserve energy.

For many animals, exercise is certainly not the key to good health. Sloths spend their lives hanging, motionless, from trees. Koalas spend most of their day asleep. In fact, our great ape ancestors are even lazier, spending 18 hours a day either resting or sleeping. 'Life is essentially a game of turning energy into kids, and every trait is tuned by natural selection to maximise the evolutionary return on each calorie spent,' Associate Professor Herman Pontzer, an anthropologist at the University of Southern California who has done much to understand this paradox, writes in *New Scientist.*

Yet humans seem to need to move. There's an enormous wealth of evidence showing the health benefits of regular exercise. Regular exercise reduces your chances of getting several types of cancer: breast (about 20 to 30 per cent), prostate (about 10 per cent), endometrial (about 23 to 29 per cent) and ovarian (about 19 per cent). It cuts your chances of death from heart problems by half. It cuts the risk of type 2 diabetes and osteoporosis. It reduces your chances of *dying early* by between 20 and 35 per cent.

Why? *Why is mindless pedalling on an exercise bike, or running in a loop, so damn good for us?* Pontzer thinks he has the answer. In a series of studies using chemically labelled water, Pontzer and his team showed the amount of energy humans use all around the world is essentially the same.[1] A sedentary video-gamer uses the same amount of energy as a hunter–gatherer, who uses the same amount of energy as a Nigerian farmer. People who are very active use only a little bit more energy than people who are not.

This is a startling fact with big implications.

When we lived as hunter–gatherers, we worked hard and were very healthy. Evidence from modern hunter-gatherers suggests almost two hours of vigorous exercise a day might be the norm. This is the lifestyle our bodies evolved to support. We spent our energy on exercise. Now we are sedentary, *but use the same amount of energy.* And all that energy needs to go somewhere. When an animal rests, much of its energy gets concentrated on accelerating wound healing, tuning up the immune system, or dealing with stress. That's good – in small doses. Your average hunter–gatherer probably only had small periods where she could sit down and heal. Modern humans have the opposite scenario. We have heaps of energy, and nothing to do with it. That, Pontzer argues, deluges our systems with energy.

A healthy immune system, overloaded with energy, becomes inflammatory. Without an outlet, the stress system becomes overloaded, leaving you stressed, anxious and unhealthy. People who are fitter are physically less prone to stress and anxiety. Exercise, Pontzer thinks, is the price we now must pay for our modern lives. We generate so much surplus energy that without working it off we become stressed and inflamed and miserable. Viewed this way, exercise is *essential,* not optional, if you want to be healthy.

And exercise is particularly good for the back. Let's go to our friends at Cochrane. In late 2021 they produced a pretty extraordinary review, pulling together data from 249 studies – a total of 24 486 people. The conclusion, when all the data was pooled: exercise does improve chronic low back pain. Pain levels go down, and so do disability levels – that is, people get their life back. The evidence suggests that, in general, it helps more than nearly everything else we do for chronic low back pain, like steroids or surgery. Exercise is medicine. And it's not just a placebo. It *beats* the placebo.

An even more exciting study was published in *Pain* in 2022.[2] The team tracked 126 people with chronic back pain for a month while wearable sensors monitored their sleep and exercise. The volunteers were given a smartphone app to register how their back was feeling and any pain flare-ups. This study is particularly cool because it could look at what was happening *before* the volunteers had a flare of their back pain – and the findings really strengthen the case for exercise. People who moved less were *more* likely to report a back pain flare the next day, while those who spent time doing gentle exercise – or even a lot of standing – seemed to be slightly protected.

This data doesn't tell us if any form of exercise is better than another – just that exercise, in general, helps. Why? One theory: it rebuilds the connection between our brain and back. Movement fires neurons in the motor cortex; the feeling of twisting and bending fires up the sensory system. 'It rewires those motor patterns. If you have an abnormal movement pattern, getting someone to move in the correct way in theory could promote a reversal,' says Rocco Cavaleri, physiotherapist and neuroscientist. 'And hopefully that could, long-term, reduce their pain.'

So exercise is the price we must pay for our modern lives, if we want to remain healthy. And it is amazingly good for our backs. But it also has an unusual feature: it changes us.

When you lift weights at the gym, or go for a jog, you're sending a signal to your body. It knows you're trying to do a physical task of which your muscles are not quite capable. So your body adapts. Your muscles thicken, new neural connections are laid down, and your strength increases. Your blood vessels and organs are strained, and so grow stronger. Exercise prompts our body to start self-repairing; without it, we grow weaker over time, particularly as we age. The same principle applies to the back. By using it, by moving it through new angles and flexing it and adding weight, it grows stronger.

The body *craves* load.

'It's only movement and loading that will get the tissues back to as healthy as they can be,' Lorimer Moseley. 'Everything is adaptable, our system will adapt. If you take the load away, it will become less strong.'

It's only natural to want to protect an injured or sore area. Many people with back pain are afraid of bending, or moving. I spent a few months refusing point-blank to lift our arthritic dog into the car because I was worried I'd hurt my back, much to the frustration of my mother. Other people jam their back muscles up tight to prevent further damage – my dad did that. He described the hell of having every muscle in his back running at 100 per cent every moment of every day, until the exhausted musculature finally collapsed in spasm.

What happens when we avoid movement or load? Our backs get *weaker*, not stronger. Without movement, back muscles atrophy, amplifying the feeling of pain when the back does move.

There are a lot of big muscles in your back. They feel pain a bit differently to other tissues. Rather than being sensitive to sharp jabs, big muscles contain sensors that look for chemical changes in the muscle caused by overuse. Try holding your hands over your head for as long as you can. Notice how sore your shoulders get. There's no tissue damage going on; your muscles are simply registering fatigue as pain. Your back muscles do exactly the same thing. Hold them tense for too long and they'll hurt. Hold them tense for months and they'll spasm.

Evidence suggests muscles that are not used often are weaker, fatigue sooner, and feel that fatigue-pain worse. Muscles that are regularly worked – it doesn't have to be in the gym, just being used for movement seems enough – are more fatigue-resistant and feel less pain. A strong back is a healthy back. *The body craves load.*

Many exercises claim to be the magic bullet for back pain. The evidence generally doesn't bear those claims out. A team from Deakin University combed through almost a hundred studies covering 5578 back pain patients treated with exercise. Their conclusion: there is no one best exercise for lower back pain. But there are several that seem to help in different ways. Pilates produced the best results in cutting pain. Running and lifting weights were best for mental health outcomes.

And stabilisation training was best for getting the back moving naturally again. 'They're active kinds of exercise where a clinician or a therapist is taking them through a program of exercise, where someone develops their confidence in movement,' Deakin University's Associate Professor Daniel Belavy tells me. 'And it helps that person to manage their fear of pain and learn that if I do this thing it isn't going to make my pain worse. It helps them to break that cycle.'

The real key, he says, is simply to get active. Exercise of nearly any form is likely helpful.

Spine surgeon Dr Michael Johnson agrees. 'I'm sure there are people who'll swear by this or that,' he told me. 'I think the basic thing is just that people need exercise. Whether that's walking, swimming, cycling, doesn't matter. Just do *some* type of exercise. And there's good evidence that people who exercise do better.'

Lastly, exercise is one of the only things that seems to really *prevent* back pain. Chris Maher and his colleagues reviewed the evidence for the *Lancet*.[3] Back braces, shoe insoles, ergonomic interventions at the office: the evidence suggests they probably don't work. But exercise, in whatever form, does work. If there's one thing you can take away from this book, it's this: exercise is magic, and both prevents and treats back pain.

Movement, strength and ballet

To see the value of exercise in action, we can look to some of the world's elite athletes: dancers.

The Australian Ballet Company has five ranks. Young dancers, fresh out of the finest training schools in Melbourne and Sydney, Moscow and New York, start in the *corps de ballet*, the ballet's chorus. If they perform well, and if their bodies hold up, they can progress, first to *coryphée* (a dancer who dances in a small group rather than the chorus or as a soloist), and then on to soloist, then to senior artist. At the top is the principal artist, the best athletes, the stars of the show. The company has just ten. For artists, becoming a principal in a world-renowned company like the Australian Ballet is to reach the pinnacle of their profession. It's something you dedicate your life to.

Ty King-Wall reached that summit. And then his back took it away from him. King-Wall is tall and blonde with green eyes and the lithe, muscular frame of a man whose job it is to make something very physically difficult look easy and effortless and beautiful. When he was 20, he herniated a disc. L4–L5, the disc that sits between the bottom two vertebrae in the back. Like many people, he found his first injury painful but manageable, and he didn't take too much time off dancing.

Every morning, the company's dancers assemble for a warm-up and technical practice session before several hours of rehearsal. As everyone went through their routines, King-Wall noticed his foot wasn't cooperating properly. It refused to rise onto demi-pointe. The nerve signals coming from it were wrong, clouded in a harsh static of pins and needles. He couldn't feel his toes. 'I thought it was just because I hadn't warmed up. But then I found every time I tried to go up on demi-pointe my leg would drop out from under me. It was a bit scary.' King-Wall didn't know it at the time, but he'd blown another disc. It was worse this time – the L5–S1 disc, which lies between the bottom vertebra and the sacrum. The disc ejected some of its jelly-like filling into his spine, putting pressure on nearby nerves and interrupting the passage of information between his foot and his brain.

That required a longer break, but again King-Wall came back, determined. He rested, then recovered and rebuilt himself, pushed through the pain to get back on stage. He thought he was OK. Until one night he was flying across the floorboards, came down hard on one leg and feet as though someone had shot him right in the calf. He somehow limped off, assuming he'd torn a calf muscle. But the ballet's medical team couldn't find any damage in the area. Eventually, they traced it back – back to the old injury at L5–S1. The disc's jelly-like filling had again started to push on his nerve roots. This time, the pain didn't go away.

Ballet dancers move between classical 'positions', each pose a word in a poem. The arabesque is considered the essence of ballet, perhaps the most beautiful and the hardest to master. Without it, a ballet dancer cannot dance. The dancer stands on one leg, then lifts the other leg behind them. The L5–S1 disc lies right at the hinge point for this movement. 'If you don't have the flexibility in your back to keep it upright, you put that disc under immense pressure,' King-Wall says. After the injury, he couldn't even come close to making the shape.

King-Wall's partner, Amber Scott – who's had her own struggles with back pain – remembers seeing him then, lost in a black cloud. 'Back pain – it really radiates to the core of your being. I could see it. It's really distressing psychologically,' she told me. 'You cannot get away from it, when you lie down or leave practice. To get rest, to sleep properly – disc problems hinder that as well.'

King-Wall thought his career was over. He readied himself to retire. Sue Mayes had other ideas. Dr Mayes is the Australian Ballet's longtime principal physiotherapist. She's a world leader in her field, caring for the dancers while also finding time to author several research papers and travel the world presenting her findings.

She's so good, the globe's best seek her out – like David Hallberg, the first ever American to become the Bolshoi Ballet's principal dancer. In 2014, after years of wringing the most out of his body at the highest pinnacle of his art, his left ankle fell apart. A botched reconstructive surgery left his ankle 'a mess', he told *Vulture* magazine.[4] After a year of failed rehab, he faced a stark choice: retire, or travel to the Antipodes to chase a miracle cure. He chose the latter, deleted all his social media accounts, retreated from the world, and handed his body over to Mayes and her team.

A dancer who could have picked any high-tech hospital or surgeon in the world to work with ended up hiding in Melbourne for 14 months, working painstakingly to rebuild his body – and his mind.

Mayes set two pillars for Hallberg's rehab. He needed to regain strength in the ankle, obviously, which he did over twice-a-day gruelling workouts. But he also needed to understand how his body processed pain, and why that process had gone wrong. 'It was important he understand that what he was feeling was exaggerated,' Mayes later told *Dance Magazine*. 'He had built up so much fear about the damage, and fear exacerbates symptoms, adding to the dysfunction.'[5]

Mayes kept her promise. She guided Hallberg's rebuild. After a three-year absence, he returned to the stage at the Metropolitan Opera House in New York, to standing ovations.

Ballet dancing puts a lot of strain on a performer's back. Female dancers are required to hyperextend their spines backwards and forwards to form graceful shapes, while the males need to lift, hold and twirl their partners above their heads. About 30 per cent of all injuries the Australian Ballet Company suffers are back injuries, Mayes tells me. These injuries can be career-ending; before Mayes got involved, a bulged disc would often push a dancer into retirement. But in the last 20 years she's worked with the dancers, she's not had one back-injury-related retirement. And zero back surgeries. 'We have never operated on a back – which I think is really important,' Mayes says.

Compared to the average desk-based worker, a dancer's chances of spinal and disc injury are high. If there was a place where physical treatments for back pain, rather than mental approaches, would be embraced, it would be among elite athletics. Yet here, right at the pinnacle of ballet, Mayes focuses on mental strength, physical resilience, and keeping everyone out of the surgeon's office.

Mayes's first tenet for dancers with back pain: no X-rays. A scan might be ordered when the medical team suspects something serious has gone wrong, but for an uncomplicated back injury, scans are off limits. 'A lot of the fear that has built up – we hear about disc prolapses, disc bulging – we're fearful that's going to happen to us, and that's going to be the end of our career. And a lot of that fear can drive dysfunction,' Mayes says. 'So we don't do much imaging for that reason. Because we know we're probably going to find something incidental that's not necessarily the source of the pain.'

Keeping an athlete out of the X-ray booth proves a hard task. Their bodies represent their livelihood, and if there's a hint of something going wrong they're keen to look under the hood. Mayes's team gently explains the research behind the decision not to scan. 'And if they're still keen to look, they need psychological counselling. Because no matter what we say, once they've seen the scan, it just sticks in their head: they have a disc bulge. And it creates so much fear. So we involve a psych to help them through these fears.'

And then Mayes gets them moving, working through a lengthy and individualised strengthening program to rebuild them stronger than ever. 'Most people get scared about injury,' she says. 'But the worst thing you can do for any injury – and particularly back pain – is stop moving.'

To rebuild King-Wall's back, Mayes needed him to

move. Even though it hurt. Because avoiding the pain, or dulling it with drugs, was never going to fix the problem. King-Wall spent a lot of time in the pool, keeping his back moving. He worked on his lower body, building the strength to support his back. He did a lot of Pilates. He visualised his spine moving gracefully. Mayes has worked with other academics on developing a program of guided visualisation for back pain, linking the soft sound of running water with an image held in the mind's eye of a river gently carving through the landscape. *This is how my spine must be*, the athletes repeat to themselves, *gentle and flexible.*

Movement and strength are the keys to healing back pain, Mayes says. They're also the key to preventing it. The body and the back need to be strong. 'But it's how they get that strength that's important,' says Mayes. Every dancer at the Australian Ballet gets an individual training program customised to their body. Back and core strength are integral. Mayes puts particular emphasis on what she refers to as 'interflexion': strength through the flex of the muscle. Building the strength to hold a single pose – like, say, a plank – is nice, but doesn't do much to protect the back, says Mayes.

All this was personally dispiriting: I'd been doing a torturous routine of planks at the gym for the last year, after reading somewhere they were the new crunch. That wasn't going to protect my back at all, Mayes told me. The back needs to be strong through its *range* of motion, she explained, particularly if you were planning to pick someone else up from the floor and spin them above your head.

Mayes's dancers do simple gym exercises: squats, Russian deadlifts, step-ups. A back was only as strong as its supporting structures, she explained, and that support started in the huge muscles below the base of the spine: the thighs and hamstrings and the gluteus maximus, the largest and strongest muscle in your body.

'The gluteus?' I ask, writing notes.

'The, uh, buttocks,' says Mayes.

The lower body and the butt form a strong base for the spine to flex. A strong base takes load off the back. They're often overlooked when people are looking to strengthen their back, but they shouldn't be – they're the supporting structure. To protect the back, Mayes prescribes exercise in general: bike riding, swimming, running. Anything at all helps. 'The bottom line is, movement is important,' she said.

If I wanted to get more technical, working at a gym on exercises that built flexible strength in my lower body, back and core would all do me well. So – squats? 'Yeah,' she said. 'We really like squats.'

Mayes's dancers have a big advantage you and I do not: they're part of an elite athletic team staffed with strength and conditioning coaches and physiotherapists. You and I have access to our local gym and a helpful but possibly not highly trained PT.

An expert can help

Talking to Mayes, and trying to build my own exercise program at the gym, I kept coming back to Shannon Noll's story. Noll had tried just this approach: he'd trained, hard. He had a freakin' six-pack! He was at the gym five days a week, focusing on his core – just like all the fitness magazines tell us to do to treat a sore back. It didn't work.

Some people might be able to build their own program that gets them out of the dark spiral of back pain. But it doesn't work for everyone. In those cases, an exercise program delivered by a highly trained expert – either a physiotherapist or an exercise physiologist – who specialises in sore backs may have a lot of value.

'We put expectations on the fitness industry that are inappropriate. People who have back pain shouldn't be going to a personal trainer,' says Tim Dettmann. 'They should be going to the health industry.'

Dettmann is a university-educated physiotherapist and director of Kieser Australia, a global company that specialises in exercise-based treatment for back pain. As we chatted, it was like listening to all my research for this book fall out of his mouth. Core exercises are overrated. Lifting with a straight back is silly. Ergonomics doesn't work. 'Surgery takes a day. Ergonomics takes $500. There's something in the psyche of people – we're always, unfortunately, looking for the quick fix. Science never has, and probably never will, support a quick fix. You need to do exercise and you need to do it for at least 12 months.'

Kieser doesn't offer a quick fix. It offers slow, progressive exercise supervised by a physiotherapist.

'When people have back pain, we know their body goes into a protection mode. The consequences of that protection mode is they become centrally sensitised – and they also start to get atrophy of the muscles they should be using,' Dettmann tells me. 'You get back pain and someone says "Don't bend your back". Wonderful short-term strategy, horrible long-term strategy. It's going to stop you having pain today. But it's going to resign you to having pain in the future. Your body's going to forget how to move. You're going to become weak and uncoordinated.'

Kieser studios have weight machines that look similar to those you might find in your local gym. But these are much more expensive, because they're much more adjustable. Most of their machines can go up and down in weight by about 450 grams. That's so little you barely feel it, Dettmann says, and allows the physiotherapists to progressively build strength in muscles that have become deconditioned.

Over 12 weeks, a person with back pain will slowly be progressed through a range of exercises to build strength in their back. The weights are raised so slowly they don't even notice they're getting stronger; before they know it, people who couldn't lift anything at all are lifting something quite heavy.

I tell him about Shannon Noll's story. Dettmann is unsurprised. 'There's no correlation between what you look like on the front and how your back performs. There will be plenty of people with aesthetically impressive bodies who have back pain,' he says. Plenty of elite athletes, like the ballet dancers we just met, have back pain. 'There's zero correlation between a six-pack and back pain,' Dettmann says.

Along with a loss of strength, many people with back pain develop a lot of fear of movement – fear of bending and twisting and lifting, worried about a spike in pain or injuring themselves seriously. But pushing, little by little, *into* this pain is a key part of the treatment. Dettmann quotes Moseley: you need to turn down the brain's protectometer. By edging into the pain, little by little, you can teach the brain that actually the tissue isn't damaged – there's nothing that needs *protecting*. A less-worried brain produces less pain. Dettmann wants his patients to become stronger, but also less fearful and more self-confident.

'I never want a patient to think I'm saying "The pain is in your head",' he tells me. 'It's not. You're not making it up. It's that your brain is amplifying the pain to try to protect you. Exercise can turn the volume down over time.'

He has one final pillar of treatment, this one also backed by evidence: a referral to a pain psychologist.

Pain psychology

Ty King-Wall had to rebuild his body. He also had to rebuild his mind. 'Initially I was quite stubborn about the mental side of things,' he says. 'I thought: I have an injury, that's why I feel pain and feel down. And once the injury's fixed, the pain will go away and I'll feel better. And it took me a little while to get – how do I say this – the idea that I could be contributing to my perception of the pain. I could be increasing my experience of the pain, through where my head was at.'

The pain was caused by the physical injury. But it was being amplified by the way he'd started to think about the pain. And it wouldn't go away until he could master both domains.

King-Wall worked with the company's psychologist, an avuncular sports doctor by the name of David Williams, who we met in Chapter 11. To get better, Williams told him, the dancer would need to separate 'the pain that was coming from the injury itself, and pain that I was contributing myself mentally through stress, anxiety, and constantly focusing on the injured area'.

'My back was definitely damaged. But it was important to acknowledge that it was on two levels, mental and physical. Accepting that I was damaged, and not placing unrealistic expectations on a miraculous recovery and being 100 per cent pain free, allowed me to stay in the moment and concentrate on what I could control,' says King-Wall 'Then the pain did start to fade.'

Williams has moved on from the ballet now, into his own private practice, where he sees private pain patients while still doing consulting work for sports clubs – he spends a lot of time with the Melbourne Demons AFL club. It's hard to think of a more different arena to ballet when it comes to dealing with back pain, I tell him. He shrugs. The treatment pathway for getting better, be it acute or chronic back pain or any other lingering pain, is much the same. It still includes an immediate referral to a psychologist.

An athlete's ability to move is central to their identity. There's an understanding in clubs now that any case of long-term pain, or restriction in the ability to physically do something, can have a major effect on a player's psyche, and that if they get stuck in a dark spiral their entire rehab can be compromised. 'If you take away the ability to move the way they're used to, it starts to challenge how they feel in the world,' says Williams. He now works with footballers to help them develop what he calls 'passive strategies' to manage pain – things like meditation, relaxation and mindfulness.

Athletes also offer an interesting case study for how a certain mindset can help us deal with pain, says Williams. 'In some of the WorkCover cases I've worked with, where pain was the central feature, you could see very quickly how the person's behaviour – willingness to move, confidence to move – had become inhibited by pain,' he says. 'In people with really strong athletic backgrounds, what I've noticed is there's a willingness to push and experience pain, and see pain as an important part of getting better. They have a conceptualisation of pain that may be very different to what you or I have.'

Footballers play through enormous amounts of pain. There's the obvious stuff, like the bone-jarring collisions that make the crowd 100 metres away wince. But there's also the less obvious stuff, like the ability to run through the burn of fatigue, to push through all the natural stops the body tries to erect and keep going in a desperate effort to win. Pain sits between where they are and where they want to be. Going towards and through the pain is the only way to win. That's something the average person could take away from a footballer, Williams reckons. Rehab from any back condition is painful, but if you can build a mentality that pain is something to endure and break through, then you get a whole new perspective on that pain. In this mindset, pain is not a signal to stop. It's a signal the body is testing its limits. And if you push through the pain, you can get stronger. You might even learn to seek the pain, because then you know whatever you're doing is working.

Psychology can help build a stronger, more resilient mindset. It can also help us directly treat back pain. The gold standard treatment for back pain, experts told me again and again, was a multidisciplinary approach, with psychology as a cornerstone. Two treatment approaches stand out for their strong scientific backing: cognitive behavioural therapy and acceptance commitment therapy. If you're seeking psychological help, ask for these treatments.

CBT, as it is known, has a strong evidence base for treating a wide range of mental illnesses, including chronic low back pain. CBT takes aim at *how* we think and behave, looking for faulty lines of logic or reasoning or unhelpful behaviours, and trying to correct them. Acceptance commitment therapy is interested in the end point of our back pain journey: returning to life. How do we fit any pain we might still have around our lives? How can we keep doing the things that matter, while finding ways around the things that cause pain to flare? The therapy involves a lot of mindfulness: accepting that things like pain intrude on our consciousness automatically, but also standing apart from them. *We are not our pain.* There's high-level evidence that acceptance commitment therapy beats both a placebo and treatment-as-usual for anxiety, depression and pain; it seems to work just as well as CBT.[6]

And now a major systematic review hot off the presses from the *BMJ* suggests these fixes work best when combined with structured exercise programs delivered by a physio.[7] On the basis of this evidence, I think if you've got long-term chronic back pain, you really, really should be looking at signing up to both a physio and a psych and getting them working together.

Pain psychologist Jess Chu works with people with back pain to help them accept a level of pain as normal. If you can come to terms with the pain, learn to slide it to the back of your mind, over time the wailing alarm will turn into a dull tone, and then eventually one you don't even notice as you go about your day-to-day life. Psychological treatments generally do not reduce chronic pain to zero out of ten. Instead, says Chu, they are designed to help us accept, cope, and return to living a good life. 'I try to be realistic. It's an ongoing thing you have to keep dealing with. It's something we just have to manage.'

Just like exercise, buy-in is crucial. You have to want to change, and embrace the work. 'The only way the patient's going to get any improvement is through things they do,' says Professor Michael Nicholas of the Pain Management Research Institute. 'They need to change their behaviour patterns that are unhelpful – the unhelpful ways they think about pain – become less depressed, change the way they think about the world.'

This means it's not enough to just go to a psych. That's a bit like going to a gym and having a personal training session. Without buy-in – without you going back all by yourself and hitting the weights regularly – you'll never get anywhere, says Nicholas.

Pain psychologists also teach self-management, helping people slowly, gradually exercise more and more, pushing through the pain and building up tolerance and resilience until it fades into the background. This process can be long and slow. 'There's no magic bullet,' says Nicholas. You need to be firm with yourself. Put a list of possible things you could do that might improve your situation down on paper, and start working through them. And give yourself a hard deadline. I'll start swimming – today. I'll see my friends – today. It's long and slow and, often, hard. It requires work and commitment, unlike the quick fixes spruiked by so many. But it does work.

'You see a definite change in people's mentality,' says Jess Chu. 'No longer do they feel like the pain is taking over their lives. They have a say in what they do. There's always going to be some limitation at times – but it's just like with money. Most people have limitations on what they can buy. It's about figuring out a budget, saving up for it, building up that resilience.'

Rebuilding the mind doesn't always have to come via a shrink. As the evidence for this approach has mounted – and the evidence for a biomechanical approach has declined – more and more physiotherapists have started combining exercise for body and brain.

Near the completion of this book, soon after the birth of my daughter, I found myself in a pub in Brunswick, drinking a beer while she gurgled happily in the stroller next to me. Like most new parents, I was totally exhausted. Alex sat down next to me, looked at the bags under my eyes, cracked a grin. 'And you're trying to write a book too?'

We can't all make good life choices. Anyway, Alex had a story for me. He'd been struggling with chronic muscle pain, and he'd run into a practitioner who'd tried on him techniques that sounded a lot like what I'd been writing about. And they'd worked.

For about ten years Alex had struggled with iliotibial band syndrome – chronic tenderness across the outside of the leg and knee. It's a classic runner's injury, and is extraordinarily painful. Alex had tried everything – massage, manipulation, stretching. Nothing worked. At his wits' end, he booked in to see an exercise physiologist, an expert in exercise-based rehab. The physiologist – Alex thought his name might have been Luke – looked him over, nodding and tutting and shaking his head. 'And then,' Alex turned to look me in the eye, 'he told me that I was totally fine. And there was nothing he could really do.

'He said the ligament I'd been trying to stretch – you could attach a metric tonne to that ligament and it wouldn't stretch at all. It's not tight, it's not damaged. It's normal. The problem is the pain, not the ligament. He told me I just had to run through it.' Alex leaned forward over his beer. 'He told me to go away and keep running, and he never wanted to see me again.' Alex sat back, shook his head. 'And so I kept running, and kept telling myself my body was fine, and slowly it went away. And I've been pain-free for years.'

Luke turns out to be Luke Postlethwaite, a disciple of Peter O'Sullivan and Lorimer Moseley, exercise physiologist and founder of The Biomechanics, a multidisciplinary clinic in Footscray. He has people with back pain walk in every day, he says. Some people come in worried after they felt a tweak or a ping in their back – have they damaged it? That's better than the poor people who've fallen into back pain's dark spiral. They turn up with three segments of their spines fused, still in pain.

Postlethwaite likes to start his back pain consultations with the same question: what would you do if you had a headache? You wouldn't spend the day in bed. In all probability, you'd go to work, and rub your temples. Your colleagues might ask if you'd had a bit too much to drink last night. Maybe it's stress. Are you drinking enough water? Now, says Postlethwaite, imagine the same scenario – but you've got back pain. You're walking with a hunch. You're not going to work. You're worrying you've done some sort of permanent damage. Two similar pains. Two different thought processes. 'The *only* difference is the location in which we experience it,' says Postlethwaite.

At the start of his career, Postlethwaite offered treatments that focused on the soft tissue: manipulation, massage, TENS machines – all the fancy tools of physiotherapy that I used to pay to have applied to my back. But over time, he's been forced to admit to himself and his patients that the evidence really doesn't support that stuff. What the evidence does show, he says, is that people can cut their pain by changing the way they think about it. 'The biggest thing we try to teach is we don't have pain nerves, we don't have pain signals. We have danger signals, and your brain interprets that with a whole bunch of other information. We treat pain as an experience.'

Key to this is pushing the message that pain doesn't mean damage. We think we're bizarrely fragile. Does it really make sense that bending over too quickly, or sleeping funny in bed, can actually damage our spines? 'Humans are so much more robust than that,' says Postlethwaite.

This is important to remember when you're exercising. Exercise often hurts. Our muscles strain; our back muscles get tired. The next morning we wake up stiff and tender. But that's not a sign of long-term damage being done. Our bodies can handle it. Remember, they *crave load*.

Really, the key tool in Postlethwaite's arsenal is just talking. Combatting those harmful ideas we have about backs. Giving people the confidence they need to get moving again, so they don't become stiff. 'We look for opportunities where their narrative doesn't meet up with current research. They say "I know it's because my posture's bad". Well, actually, there's no association between posture and back pain. Or "I've had a scan and I've got a disc bulge". Well, so do 80 per cent of 20 year olds.

'Statistically, the odds are in your favour. Most serious spinal conditions don't hurt that much. Think about paraplegia or quadriplegia. It doesn't hurt. You lose sensation. If you've got back and leg pain, the good chance is it's probably OK.'

Manual therapies

I spent a lot of time over the years face down on the couch, having my back and spine worked on. Dad's physio tried all sorts of things on my sore back: ultrasound (conducted not by the physio himself but by his secretary), spinal massage, even traction – using a winch to slowly pull my hips away from my ribcage, lengthening my spine. I later told another physio about it. She did a double-take. 'That is some seriously old-school stuff.'

Before that, when I was younger, it was Mum's chiropractor, who pulled at my neck and hit me with a clicker and twisted me till I cracked. Did these treatments work? I found myself wondering years later.

Directly manipulating the spine is called manual therapy. And it's ancient. Hippocrates, the father of medicine, promoted manual spinal manipulation and traction. Jesus lays on his hands on those who are to be healed. Today it's offered by physiotherapists and chiropractors. Does it work? To an extent. Our friends at Cochrane reviewed studies of spinal manipulation, as performed by chiropractors, and compared that with the broad range of treatments delivered by physiotherapists. The results: both kinds of treatment worked about the same. Neither was better or worse than the other.

So, if you're seeing a chiro or a physio to get rubbed and adjusted and you feel like it's working, the evidence suggests you can happily keep going. *However.* While they offer a similar treatment, there's a big difference in the *approach* these two professions take that's worth talking about. Physiotherapy is meant to be evidence-based. That's why you've met so many physiotherapists in this book, beavering away at clinical trials and research papers. A physio will offer manual therapy, but so much more; perhaps most valuable, they tend to focus a lot on exercise, helping you design a movement program that will get you heading towards feeling better without overdoing it and hurting yourself.

Chiropractic is not based on hard evidence; it is alternative medicine. Its provenance dates back to 18 September 1895, when magnetic healer DD Palmer shoved the vertebrae of a deaf janitor in downtown Davenport, Iowa, and apparently restored his hearing. Palmer claimed he'd discovered a cure to life's maladies. He termed his misaligned vertebrae 'subluxation' (a word borrowed from craft healers), a shift of the vertebrae in the spine that can irritate nearby nerves. These misalignments can be caused by a physical injury, or something more benign, chiros claim: chemical exposure, dehydration, stress.

Palmer believed these misaligned vertebrae altered the natural flow of energy through the body. BJ Palmer, his son and a key figure in the early development of chiropractic, went further. He believed subluxation was the root of nearly all contagious diseases, like smallpox.

Does subluxation exist? Is it really the root of back pain? You may be surprised to learn, given its centrality to the practice, that many modern chiropractors are sceptical. There are now a number of chiropractors tenured to universities as academic staff; it's hard for them to ignore outright quackery altogether. A review of the evidence for subluxation by several chiropractors found there simply was no evidence to say one way or the other.

This leaves chiros in a tricky position, I think. There's good evidence spinal manipulation does somewhat help with back pain. But much of the profession is thoroughly unscientific – hence the strong overlap between chiropractors and anti-vax activists. Chiro researchers even had to go so far as to issue a joint statement warning the public that, despite what many chiros claimed, spinal manipulation could not boost immunity.[8] And let's remember the evidence: how we *think* about our backs has a big effect on how they feel – which is why having chiros do some sort of 'scan' and then give patients a report noting extreme spinal dysfunction, with the problematic vertebrae highlighted in red, is so *bad*.

Some chiros may not be interested in subluxation as a cause of disease. Some may only want to perform spinal manipulation, knowing it works as well as the alternatives. 'That would be perfectly fine,' says Chris Maher. 'Unfortunately, most don't. They end up offering their patients all sorts of weird shit.'

Pain education

In the middle of the desert, surrounded by the picked-clean bones of unlucky animals, stand three dirty metal cages. The cages are big, perhaps 4 metres tall, and divided horizontally by a platform. From the centre platform jut two dozen wooden pegs of varying length and width, the thinnest the diameter of a Coca-Cola bottle. From the floor below, another series of small pegs rises to meet them, like stalagmites and stalactites. Firelight plays over the structures, and the night vanishes the desert behind them. They look … well, they look like torture chambers.

And there, in the middle of one of the chambers, hands grasping the pegs above her, feet balanced on the thin wood beneath, stands Hayley Leake. She squats, really; by this stage of the challenge the central platform has been lowered so far she has no choice. Leake has been squatting like this for five hours now. Five hours of torture. She's enduring it just like she's endured every challenge up until this point: with total calm, total composure, total zen-like focus.

Across from her, her opponent is starting to waver. Her face screws up. She breathes deeply, opens her eyes, looks around, readjusts her grip. There are tears in her eyes. She stares at Leake, trying to tell how long she has left. Leake stays calm, focuses on her task.

Nope. Leake's competitor can't do it. She crushes her nose into her arm, and then she's done, calling to the TV program's staff to get her off this thing. The TV cameras cut back to Leake, watching her opponent collapse. She's still calm in this moment of triumph. You get the sense she could have done a few more hours. Maybe that's why her opponent waved the white flag.

Leake is one of the most dominant ever contestants on *Australian Survivor*, the game show in which players compete in tests of physical and mental endurance in the middle of the wilderness.

She came into the competition as a scientist. If she was going to win, the expectation was she'd need to outwit the other players. She ended it as winner of the most immunity challenges ever by an Australian player. Leake's secret? Immense physical and mental toughness. A competitiveness and fiery will to win. A razor-sharp intellect. And, as a physiotherapist and chronic pain researcher at Neuroscience Research Australia, someone with a working knowledge of the science of pain.

'I tell myself "If I stand here for ten hours, what's the worst that's going to happen?" I'm not going to break a bone. My nerves are going to be fine. I'm not going to do any permanent damage. What about my muscles and ligaments? Unless I twist and fall off, I have no risk,' Leake tells me. 'I could reevaluate how threatening it was, because I felt confident in my body tissue. I could reiterate "This is painful, but it's not harmful, so I can hold on".'

As we've seen, pain is not a hard mechanical signal but a *decision* made by the brain in response to its environment. What that means – the really exciting bit – is if you can convince the brain to change its decision, you can cut pain.

The evidence, remarkably, really does suggest this approach – formalised by Lorimer Moseley and others in a program called 'pain science education' – works. A meta-review of 12 randomised controlled trials, covering

755 people in total, and published in the leading journal *Pain* in 2019, shows learning about how pain *really* works really does lead to small improvements in pain levels and improve people's ability to go about their lives.[9] Another meta-review published in the *European Journal of Pain* found similar effects.[10] The effects are small, but remember, you can stack them on top of a structured exercise program – rebuilding mind and body at the same time.

Moseley started working in the space after an epiphany while working as a young physio evaluating a government-run pain management program. The program included an early form of pain education, teaching people the basics of modern pain science. 'As a rule, they were having this rapid reduction in disability. But they had no change in pain,' Moseley says. 'I remember thinking [that] according to my understanding of biology, this makes no sense. And then I noticed a lot of them were saying things like "Oh, it was a great program. But it wasn't really for me, because I have real pain". They were convinced the program was for people who think they have pain when they don't. What really struck me about that was these people, after an intensive pain management program, were still of the view that other people thought their pain wasn't real. So what I started doing, clinically, was focusing on that.'

First, Moseley spent time persuading his patients he really did believe them. They *were* in pain. And then he showed them the science explaining how you can have pain without tissue damage. He showed them how the nervous system was wound up into a state of high agitation in chronic pain.

'They'd come back to the next appointment and often

say "I'm feeling heaps better, whatever you did". And I didn't do anything,' Moseley says. Intrigued, he ran a series of clinical trials testing out pain education. They produced small but meaningful – and side-effect-free – reductions in pain.

'OK,' I say, holding up my hand. 'This seems odd to me – that simply being taught how pain works would actually have a measurable effect on your pain experience. Why do you think it helps people? What's the mechanism?'

'Yeah,' says Moseley. Good question. 'We don't know what the mechanism is, to be honest. But we have pretty justifiable theoretical pathways.' The brain is constantly making decisions: am I hungry? Am I tired? Am I in danger? If it decides it's in danger, it produces pain. Pain education gets into the middle of that process by teaching the brain the body is no longer in danger – even though it feels like it is.

'Pain is fundamentally dependant on meaning. The same load on your back might cause pain if you're at work and no pain if you're playing golf. *Same load*,' says Moseley. 'It's all about: what does this mean for me? As long as pain means damage, your system is going to keep winding up. But if we can convince people the modern understanding of pain is [that] back pain does not mean chronic damage, if we can convince people of that, their pain should cut. Because the brain is now thinking "I'm getting these signals, but there's no point in protecting my back". The brain is processing these signals differently.'

Moseley's pain education program is offered by a wider and wider number of physiotherapists and psychologists – and now even hospitals and pharmacists. If this intrigues you – and the neuroscience is fascinating just of itself – you can find a practitioner at www.painrevolution.org/connect/ expert.

Pain education seems promising. But what if you could supercharge it? That's the idea behind a treatment being tested by Rocco Cavaleri and Simon Summers at a Western Sydney University lab: stimulate the brain to boost the effect of treatment.

Summers and Cavaleri are testing out two forms of non-invasive brain stimulation. The first uses a handheld magnet to manipulate the currents of electricity that run through your brain; the second places small electrodes across the scalp and passes a gentle current of electricity through the head.

So wired, the people in the trial are given exercise therapy or pain education – with the hope the stimulation will boost the effectiveness of the treatments. 'You're basically priming the brain,' says Cavaleri. 'I think it definitely has potential. Scientists will never ever say anything works. But the technique definitely has potential.'

Cognitive functional therapy

What if you took the best parts of pain education and exercise-based rehabilitation, two things we know work, and really dialled them up to 11? You'd have a program called cognitive functional therapy – being tested right now by back pain scientist Mark Hancock and anti-posture evangelist Peter O'Sullivan.

CFT is extremely individualised. Every patient in their clinical trial is individually assessed; there's a questionnaire about pain beliefs (and pain myths), and a physio assessment of how much a person is protecting their back. Over the next three months everyone in the trial gets seven sessions with the physio. But there won't be any massages or spinal manipulation. It's all about education, dispelling myths, and gradually rebuilding confidence. 'The main differences with this approach is, one, it focuses very much on function, on getting people back doing activities they want to do; and two, it's very much coming at the large range of individual factors that can be contributing to someone's back pain,' says Hancock.

The idea is that back pain has multiple causes: fear about damage to the spine, which leads to overprotection and a back held stiff, which eventually leads to not moving at all. You need to treat all them at once. A little bit of information, myth-busting, building confidence in the back without needing to worry about posture or bracing the core.

'In early trials, the responses have been really positive – that's why we've got funding from the government. The effects have been larger than in many back pain trials, and they seem to be more sustained,' Hancock says, and sends me a few papers to prove his point. The most promising, a randomised controlled trial conducted in Bergen, Norway, *halved* the disability score for 121 patients. Patients given standard exercise therapy improved less than half as much. These are very large changes in back pain land – you can see why Hancock and O'Sullivan are excited. (As of writing, Hancock's trial was still awaiting publication in a scientific journal.)

CFT has three steps. First, there's an interview and education session called 'making sense of pain'. Then there's a movement session called 'graded exposure with control'. And you work on developing healthy lifestyle habits. 'We try to dispel these myths. The back is strong, it's safe to relax, slouch, bend and lift without protecting it,' O'Sullivan tells me.

When O'Sullivan meets a patient for the first time, he likes to start with an open-ended question. 'Tell me your story,' he'll say, rather than 'show me your charts'. By looking at their narrative, he can quickly come to grips with how his patient feels about their problem, and all the fears and beliefs they have layered on top of the pain. Then, when they've told him what postures and movements cause the most pain, he'll ask them to stand, and start moving them through those very postures. O'Sullivan will often have them do simple breathing exercises to control their stress and learn to relax.

O'Sullivan calls them 'guided behavioural experiments'. Holding the patient by the hand, he will let them test the limits of what they can do. Typically, everyone finds they can do a lot more than they think they can – and without hurting their backs. O'Sullivan wants his patients to feel the gulf between how much pain they are *expecting* when they twist and bend and how much they really feel. 'It creates prediction-error,' he says. And when the brain realises it is wrong, it's forced to start rewiring itself.

Significant reductions in pain are often reported, right here at the start of the process, O'Sullivan says. O'Sullivan wants his patients to take away two key things. One: moving and loading the spine without protection is safe. Two: pain responses can be controlled. O'Sullivan tells me his patients often experience the most relief just from dropping their defences. Worried about doing further damage to an already stuffed spine, many people hold everything stiff. 'It's like clenching your fist around a sore wrist,' says O'Sullivan. 'Clenching your back adds more load to your back. If it's sensitive, you're just making it more sensitive. And then people become fearful, so they clench more. It creates a vicious cycle.' Just relaxing, moving, and realising that it won't mean everything falls apart, can bring enormous relief.

O'Sullivan puts me on to one of his patients, Matt. Matt worked as an anaesthetic technician at a hospital in Western Australia. One day, as he was helping anaesthetise a 206-kilogram woman, she slumped off her stretcher and rolled onto him, crushing him. He felt his spine compress, and pain shot down his leg.

Initially, the pain wasn't too bad, and after a few days off he was able to return to work. But it never went away, and over the weeks that followed became worse. His GP booked him in for an MRI, which showed one torn disc and another bulging out of alignment. He received an epidural injection, with no relief. So he had three more. 'They tried different ways of doing it, different drugs. Then I had a facet joint injection. The pain was still there – it was intensifying,' he says.

MRI, opioids, injections, no improvement – Matt was being sucked into the dark vortex of chronic back pain. The next step was surgery on the damaged disc. 'There was still no change,' he says.

He went to see another surgeon, who tutted over yet another MRI of his spine. The procedure was right, he told Matt, but the original surgeon had missed his target. *This* part needed to go. He went under the knife again. 'Again, no change.'

As I took notes, I was noting at the back of my mind how much work Matt had had done to his spine. Multiple injections, each of which carries a risk of complication, and then two major surgeries to remove parts of his spine. He sounded like walking scar tissue. He went and saw a third surgeon, who told him spinal fusion was his best option, and booked him in. Matt went back to his GP, doped to the eyeballs on opioids (he was taking 15 a day), in pain, a shell of a man.

His GP called O'Sullivan. Would he consider taking a look at Matt? the GP asked. She was worried he was at risk of killing himself. In Matt's first session at O'Sullivan's clinic, the physio dropped a pen on the floor. 'Pick it up,' he said. Matt looked at him like he was mad. 'I'd been told by other doctors not to bend, not to pick any weight up over one kilogram,' he says. 'He got me doing these breathing exercises. He said breathe in, and as you breathe out, just lean forward with your knees bent and *pick up the pen*.'

O'Sullivan was right there with him, holding him by the arm. 'This isn't going to damage your back. You're capable of doing this.' Matt looked down. The pen glimmered on the carpet. He breathed in deeply, one last time, and then pushed the air from his lungs, and bent slowly towards the pen. And he made it. All the way down, and all the way back up. He looked into O'Sullivan's face, terror-sweat beading on his forehead, stunned. 'I picked it up.' He still sounds shocked. 'For the first time in two years, I had a smile on my face. He asked me how it felt, and I said to him, "Not bad".'

Harris had damaged his spine, rupturing one disc and

herniating another. He had degenerated discs, and a disc bulge. But his spinal damage was indistinguishable from that of 60 to 80 per cent of the population his age, O'Sullivan later told me. And they did not have back pain.

As I finished this chapter, I re-read O'Sullivan's quotes from our interview. He was speaking about Matt, but really his advice could apply to almost anyone with back pain.

'What you see on a scan often doesn't correlate well with what a person feels,' he told me. 'Matt thought his back was stuffed – he was highly disabled, fearful, distressed tense, inactive and he saw no way out.

'I never believed that his pathology was the driver, because as soon as I got him to relax, move, get active, strong, back to work etc., he got much less pain. Through experiencing this, he understood his back wasn't stuffed – and that he could get back to living. That's what's healthy for backs.'

Remember Jess, my best friend's partner – the one with chronic back pain, who got such good relief from James McAuley's trial? As the book was nearly finished, we got back in touch. She had more to fill me in on, she said. McAuley's trial had been good, but she wasn't pain-free. But what it really did, she said, was open the door to a different kind of treatment. Energised by her successes, Jess wanted to build on them.

She signed up for a pain management program at Royal North Shore Hospital. Two weeks of full-time sessions run by a doctor, physio and psych. She'd spend a few hours every day meditating, a few hours doing exercise, and a few hours on pain education. The whole program was based on knowledge, she says: the more knowledge you have about your pain, the better you're able to cut it and recover from it.

'These days my back pain is very low and occasionally nil, and it doesn't really impact my day-to-day life,' she tells me. 'I'd say I no longer have chronic back pain. Which is insane, to think how far I've come.'

As I put the final, finishing touches on this book, O'Sullivan got back in touch. He had the trial results, he said, and they were enormously exciting – even transformative. When I looked at the data, published in top medical journal the *Lancet*, it quickly became clear O'Sullivan was right.[11]

The large randomised controlled trial of cognitive functional therapy found the treatment halved the level of disability that patients with chronic low back pain experienced and reduced their average pain levels by about 35 per cent. And the treatment effect seemed to last for at least a year – hell, on O'Sullivan's data, it looked to be getting stronger over time, perhaps as people's confidence in their backs grew.

I called McAuley – who wasn't involved in the trial, and who I figured would be a good independent evaluator – and he was effusive. 'These give a real, new, meaningful improvement to patients – and, really importantly, it's sustained. We never see that in standard treatments of back pain.'

I called O'Sullivan, almost giddy. Here was proof – proof that all the ideas O'Sullivan and Maher and McAuley and Moseley had been working on actually worked. Proof that you really could change the way people think about back pain and then change their pain experience. O'Sullivan sounded as giddy as I did. He couldn't agree more, he told me.

Chris Maher was somewhat more restrained. The trial was well done, and the results could be trusted, but we shouldn't read them as interpretation O'Sullivan's treatment was better than McAuley's (both are, in my view, very similar therapies). But the key, he said – and McAuley agrees – is that we now have two trials testing the ideas in this book and both finding they work.

Now, the challenge was implementation. Finally, we had something that worked really well and was safe. O'Sullivan's crew are now working frantically to get it in the hands of patients. At the moment few physios offer the program, but a (growing) list is being kept at https://www.restorebackpain.com/research-team.

'We've got a job to do,' O'Sullivan tells me. 'We have to change the story on back pain. We have to change the way we treat people. We have to become fearless.'

Conclusion

I'd kept Dad updated as I wrote this book. Calls late at night to discuss my latest discovery or pull apart some new idea. Dad was excited. His son was writing a book – and it was about him! My plan was to assemble all my data and ideas and present them to him, as a sort of conclusion to this book.

But Dad was two steps in front of me. While I was trying to understand his journey, he was embarking on a new one.

After finishing up his role at the ABC in Adelaide, Dad headed to Papua New Guinea to work for the broadcaster's International Development division, training local journalists – a rather terrifying prospect for me, as PNG is one of the more dangerous developing nations in the world. Dad loved it, of course, regaling me with tales of attempted carjackings and house burglaries. The former foreign correspondent was in his element.

And while working there, Dad met another Australian expat, who'd spent years struggling with a sore back. They bonded over pain, treatments, doctor stories. By this stage Dad was in good health, his back only cramping up in times of extreme stress. His new friend was at the other end of the dark spiral – and heading down. His life was punctuated with consistent, frightfully painful back spasms.

The pair lost touch for a while, and then reunited. The conversation picked up where it left off, as it does with old friends. How's your back? Good, both men answered. Independently, both men had come to the same conclusion: the old treatments weren't working, and the best, safest way to treat chronic back pain is by targeting the brain.

Dad's friend had worked with several experts and came across the same ideas I did: pain did not mean damage. Fear needed to be overcome, stress reduced. The brain needed to be retrained.

Dad listened to his friend, and he thought about my book. And he started to believe.

'It was a bit of peer pressure. It was an approach to thinking differently. Most importantly, he was a person I trusted,' Dad tells me over a glass of pinot.

'I started to think to myself: OK, maybe it's not about injury, not about a physical or mechanical threat – maybe it's something else. I wanted something else, I was willing to listen, and gradually I was able to change my mindset.'

Big changes take time, and then often seem to happen all at once. Dad's epiphany was in the streets of Port Moresby. He'd just taken a large sum of cash out of a bank.

'It's hot, I'm isolated, and I had a lot of money in my pocket,' he says. 'And Port Moresby is one of the world's most dangerous places. And as I was walking toward the bank, my back went into spasm.'

Here it was, the moment that had haunted Dad's life for years – the extreme twisting spasm of pain.

Dad pauses, sips his wine. 'And then I breathed through it. I breathed *through* it. And I got rid of the spasm. I went into the bank, and it never came back.'

I know I live with a risk of chronic back pain. There's a strong genetic component. Considering Dad had it and I've had a long history of sharp back pain, my risk is higher than others'. The number of scary stories from people who've struggled with it for years does worry me.

But risk is just that: risk. It means there's a chance, not a guarantee. Every time I drive a car I take a risk. Every time I leave the house I take a risk. And from what I've learnt about back pain, the worst thing I can do is worry about it and stop living my life.

The evidence strongly suggests, I think, that our backs are strong and capable. They can lift great weights. Sure, they get old, but they don't often crumble. Bad posture – mine is atrocious – isn't a big risk. And there's another side to the coin. The key to healing from back pain, it seems, is the thing we're so often afraid of: movement. The body craves movement. The back craves load. We're built to move. A bit like how sharks can't breathe if they stop swimming, we can't be healthy unless we're moving. The only thing we have to fear is fear itself.

So I've resolved to move. For years I was tentative with lifting big loads at the gym, worried about hurting my back. I'm not so worried now. I've got a personal trainer and we're gradually increasing the loads through my back with deadlifts and squats. With that strength comes confidence. My body can handle this. My spine is strong.

The mental side is just as important. We need to get confident with taking on a bit of back pain every so often, understanding that it's pretty normal – we demand a lot of our backs, and sometimes they get tired. My back hurts sometimes. And now I try really hard to just shrug my shoulders and get moving. A bit of back pain is normal. When we start overthinking it, overmedicalising it, that's when the problems really start.

A few months ago, on a waterskiing trip with my extended family, I came off my skis and plunged, hard, into a brown river. The pain was sharp and acute – I felt like I'd busted a disc – and all the muscles of my back stiffened. It was all I could do to drag myself up into the boat and lie, grimacing, on the wet deck.

The next day I woke in a lot of back pain, pain that got worse when I moved. In the past I would have fretted about the pain and spent much of the day in bed or lying down on an exercise mat. Then I would have been worried about the injury for a month.

Not any more. I knew it was extremely unlikely I'd done any actual damage to my spine – and I'd soon know if I had. So I started pushing at the pain. I got up and stretched, gently, into the pain, rounding my back, demanding my frozen muscles move. It hurt! But the next time, it got easier. And over a week, it got easier and easier still, as I moved my muscles – kick-starting the healing process with lots of fresh blood – and convinced my mind that I wasn't damaged. By the end of the week, I was pain-free.

If we accept the evidence that back pain may be being driven in part by *belief*, by the way we think about and frame pain in our backs – well, part of the solution is going to be social. Changing the way we think about our backs. Changing the way we talk about them. Not freaking out when pain rears its head. When a colleague comes in with a sore back, treating it as an annoyance rather than a major problem. Seeking solutions that treat our bodies as complex, living, growing organisms that require a little stress, a little load for peak health – not as machines with readily replaceable parts.

Change the conversation, and we might be able to change back pain.

Acknowledgments

A book like this relies enormously on generosity – from people with back pain willing to tell their stories, from surgeons taking time out of their busy operating rooms, and from scientists painstakingly explaining the evidence.

I am enormously indebted and grateful to everyone who spoke to me for this book and helped me build this narrative. In particular, I'm grateful to the many people who gave up hours of their time to speak to me – and then read my copy and checked it was accurate.

A few specific people are deserving of even more thanks. Chris Maher has done more than almost anyone to see this book published – supportive of the idea from the start, full of wisdom and advice, always taking time out of his busy schedule to answer my many questions and, when the time finally came to get the manuscript published, author of an extremely supportive letter to back it. Australian science is lucky to have him.

Big thanks also need to go to James McAuley – who started me down this journey – Peter O'Sullivan, Michael Johnson, Ashish Diwan and Lorimer Moseley, all whom gave up a lot of time to get this book into its final form. Thank you.

Harriet McInerney, my publisher at NewSouth, was one of the first people to believe I could actually write a book. And then, when I said we should do back pain, she actually listened to me and bought into the project. I'm grateful for her faith, and for the faith of my agents Lyn Tranter and Karen Colston at Australian Literary Management. Tricia Dearborn's extremely diligent editing is responsible for this book being readable rather than a mess.

I also want to thank everyone who read the manuscript and provided feedback and advice, in particular Melissa Mack, Patrick Owen and Kyle Sheldrick.

This book is about my dad, and would not have been possible – obviously – without his support and enthusiasm. Thanks for everything, Dad.

Lastly, sitting down to write your first book is a leap of faith in yourself. But the one person whose faith in me has always been unshakable is Caroline Zielinski. Without her constant encouragement and belief, this project truly would have been impossible. Love you, Caroline.

Notes

Introduction: The curse of a 'bad back'

1. Australian Institute of Health and Welfare. (2019). 'Back problems' (Cat. no. PHE 231). Canberra: AIHW, <www.aihw.gov.au/reports/chronic-musculoskeletal-conditions/back-problems>.

2. Hurwitz, EL, Randhawa, K, Yu, H, Côté, P & Haldeman, S. (2018). 'The Global Spine Care Initiative: A summary of the global burden of low back and neck pain studies'. *European Spine Journal* (vol. 27, no. S6, pp. 796–801).

1 The extent of the problem

1. Balagué, F, Mannion, AF, Pellisé, F & Cedraschi, C. (2012). 'Non-specific low back pain', *Lancet* (vol. 379, no. 9814, pp. 482–491).

2. Balagué et al. 'Non-specific low back pain'.

3. 'Low back and neck pain tops US health spending'. *Institute for Health Metrics and Evaluation*, 26 February 2020, <www.healthdata.org/news-release/low-back-and-neck-pain-tops-us-health-spending>.

4. Wu, A, March, L, Zheng, X, Huang, J, Wang, X, Zhao, J, Blyth, FM, Smith, E, Buchbinder, R & Hoy, D. (2020). Global low back pain prevalence and years lived with disability from 1990 to 2017: Estimates from the Global Burden of Disease Study 2017. *Annals of Translational Medicine* (vol. 8, no. 6, pp. 299–299).

5. Briggs, AM & Buchbinder, R. (2009). 'Back pain: A national health priority area in Australia?' *Medical Journal of Australia* (vol. 190, no. 9).

6. Craig, A, O'Meley, P & Carter, P. (2019). 'The need for greater reporting of medical device incidents', *EMJ Innovation* (vol. 3, no. 1, pp. 56–63).

7. O'Connell, NE, Ferraro, MC, Gibson, W, Rice, AS, Vase, L, Coyle, D & Eccleston, C. (2021). Implanted spinal neuromodulation interventions for chronic pain in adults. *Cochrane Database of Systematic Reviews* (vol. 2022, no. 4).

8. Weiss, M & Mohr, H. 'Spinal-cord stimulators help some patients, injure others', *AP News*, 27 November 2018, <apnews.com/article/wv-state-wire-us-news-ap-top-news-sc-state-wire-health-86ba45b0a4ad44 3fad1214622d13e6cb>.

9   Sullivan, T. 'Medtronic settles $2.8 million off-label suit over neurostimulator promotion', *Policy & Medicine*, 5 May 2018, <www.policymed.com/2015/02/medtronic-settles-with-doj-for-28-million-to-resolve-false-claims-act-allegations-related-to-spinal.html>.

10 Atkinson, L, Sundaraj, SR, Brooker, C, O'Callaghan, J, Teddy, P, Salmon, J, Semple, T & Majedi, PM. (2011). 'Recommendations for patient selection in spinal cord stimulation', *Journal of Clinical Neuroscience: Official Journal of the Neurosurgical Society of Australasia* (vol. 18, no. 10, pp. 1295–302).

11 Hara, S, Andresen, H, Solheim, O, Carlsen, SM, Sundstrøm, T, Lønne, G, Lønne, VV, Taraldsen, K, Tronvik, EA, Øie, LR, Gulati, AM, Sagberg, LM, Jakola, AS, Solberg, TK, Nygaard, ØP, Salvesen, ØO & Gulati, S. (2022). 'Effect of spinal cord burst stimulation vs placebo stimulation on disability in patients with chronic radicular pain after lumbar spine surgery', *JAMA* (vol. 328, no. 15, p. 1506).

12 Ferraro, MC, Gibson, W, Rice, ASC, Vase, L, Coyle, D & O'Connell, NE. (2022). 'Spinal cord stimulation for chronic pain', *Lancet Neurology* (vol. 21, no. 5, p. 405).

13 Choi, CQ. 'Bone density drop in modern humans linked to less physical activity'. *Livescience.Com*, 23 December 2014, <www.livescience.com/49236-bone-density-human-evolution.html>.

14 Waddell, G. (2004). *The Back Pain Revolution*. 2nd edn. Edinburgh: Churchill Livingstone, p. 143.

15 Mense, S. (2008). 'Muscle pain: Mechanisms and clinical significance', *Deutsches))rzteblatt International* (vol. 105, no. 12, pp. 214–19).

16 'Twists and turns of the human spine'. *ABC Radio National*, 7 January 2017, <www.abc.net.au/radionational/programs/archived/bodysphere/the-human-spine/7902472>.

17 Gibbons, A. 'Human evolution: Gain came with pain', *Science.org*, 16 February 2013, <www.science.org/content/article/human-evolution-gain-came-pain>.

18 Weber, J & Pusch, CM. (2008). 'The lumbar spine in Neanderthals shows natural kyphosis'. *European Spine Journal* (vol. 17, suppl. 2, pp. 327–30).

19 Choi. 'Bone density drop in modern humans linked to less physical activity.

20 Burnett, A, Beard, A & Netto, K. (2016).'Back stress and assistance exercises in weightlifting'. *ISBS – Conference Proceedings Archive*.

21 Aasa, U, Svartholm, I, Andersson, F & Berglund, L. (2016). 'Injuries among weightlifters and powerlifters: A systematic review'. *British Journal of Sports Medicine* (vol. 51, no. 4, pp. 211–19).

2   You can't slip a disc

1   Edgar, M. (2007). 'The nerve supply of the lumbar intervertebral disc'. *Journal of Bone and Joint Surgery. British Volume* (vol. 89, no. 9, pp. 1135–39).

2   Bourne, ND & Reilly, T. (1991). 'Effect of a weightlifting belt on spinal shrinkage'. *British Journal of Sports Medicine* (vol. 25, no. 4, pp. 209–12).

3   Ropper, AH & Zafonte, RD. (2015). 'Sciatica'. *New England Journal of Medicine* (vol. 372, no. 13, pp. 1240–48).

4   Gibson, JA & Waddell, G. (2007). 'The effects of surgical treatments for individuals with "slipped" lumbar discs'. *Cochrane, Back and Neck Group.*

5   Takada, E, Takahashi, M & Shimada, K. (2001). 'Natural history of lumbar disc hernia with radicular leg pain: Spontaneous MRI changes of the herniated mass and correlation with clinical outcome'. *Journal of Orthopaedic Surgery* (vol. 9, no. 1, pp. 1–7).

6   Chiu, C-C, Chuang, T-Y, Chang, K-H, Wu, C-H, Lin, P- & Hsu, W-Y. (2014). 'The probability of spontaneous regression of lumbar herniated disc: A systematic review'. *Clinical Rehabilitation* (vol. 29, no. 2, pp. 184–195).

3   Disc degeneration – not a problem

1   Battié, MC, Videman, T, Kaprio, J, Gibbons, LE, Gill, K, Manninen, H, Saarela, J & Peltonen, L. (2009). 'The Twin Spine Study: Contributions to a changing view of disc degeneration'. *Spine Journal* (vol. 9, no. 1, pp. 47–59).

2   Brinjikji, W, Luetmer, PH, Comstock, B, Bresnahan, BW, Chen, LE, Deyo, RA, Halabi, S, Turner, JA, Avins, AL, James, K, Wald, JT, Kallmes, DF & Jarvik, JG. (2014). 'Systematic literature review of imaging features of spinal degeneration in asymptomatic populations'. *American Journal of Neuroradiology* (vol. 36, no. 4, pp. 811–16).

3   Uman, LS. (2011). 'Systematic reviews and meta-analyses'. *Journal of the Canadian Academy of Child and Adolescent Psychiatry* (vol. 20, no. 1, pp. 57–59).

4   Lynch, ME, Craig, KD & Peng, PWH. (eds). (2010). *Clinical Pain Management.* 1st edn, Wiley.

5   Horga, LM, Henckel, J, Fotiadou, A, Di Laura, A, Hirschmann, AC, Lee, R & Hart, AJ. (2021). 'What happens to the lower lumbar spine after marathon running: A 3.0 T MRI study of 21 first-time marathoners'. *Skeletal Radiology* (vol. 51, no. 5, pp. 971–80).

6   Belavý, DL, Quittner, MJ, Ridgers, N, Ling, Y, Connell, D & Rantalainen, T. (2017). 'Running exercise strengthens the intervertebral disc'. *Scientific Reports* (vol. 7, no. 1).

7   'Shock over disc degeneration in 10-year olds – but are disc abnormalities in this age group surprising?' (2004). *The Back Letter* (vol. 19, no. 1, p. 1).

8   Sääksjärvi, S, Kerttula, L, Luoma, K, Paajanen, H & Waris, E. (2020). 'Disc degeneration of young low back pain patients'. *Spine* (vol. 45, no. 19, pp. 1341–47).

9   Waddell, Gordon. (2004). *The Back Pain Revolution*. 2nd edn. Edinburgh: Churchill Livingstone, p. 46.

10   Waddell. (2004). *The Back Pain Revolution*, p. 46.

11   Brown, T. (1828). 'On irritation of the spinal nerves'. *Glasgow Medical Journal* (vol. 1, no. 2, pp. 131–60).

12   Waddell. (2004). *The Back Pain Revolution*, p. 47.

13   Waddell. (2004). *The Back Pain Revolution*, p. 8.

14   Parisien, RC & Ball, PA. (1998). 'Historical perspective – William Jason Mixter (1880–1958): Ushering in the "dynasty of the disc"'. *Spine* (vol. 23, no. 21, p. 2363).

15   Mixter, WJ & Barr, JS. (1934). 'Rupture of the intervertebral disc with involvement of the spinal canal'. *New England Journal of Medicine* (vol. 211, no. 5, pp. 210–15).

16   Waddell. (2004). *The Back Pain Revolution*, p. 51.

17   Mixter, WJ & Ayer, JB. (1935). 'Herniation or rupture of the intervertebral disc into the spinal canal: Report of thirty-four cases'. *New England Journal of Medicine* (vol. 213, no. 9, pp. 385–93).

18   Carragee, E, Alamin, T, Cheng, I, Franklin, T & Hurwitz, E. (2006). 'Does minor trauma cause serious low back illness?' *Spine* (vol. 31, no. 25, pp. 2942–49).

19   Mixter & Ayer. (1935). 'Herniation or rupture of the intervertebral disc into the spinal canal'.

20   Key, JA. (1945). 'Intervertebral disk lesions are the most common cause of low back pain with or without sciatica'. *Annals of Surgery* (vol. 121, no. 4, pp. 534–39).

21   Waddell. (2004). *The Back Pain Revolution*, p. 51.

22   Lutz, GK, Butzlaff, M & Schultz-Venrath, U. (2003). 'Looking back on back pain: Trial and error of diagnoses in the 20th century'. *Spine* (vol. 28, no. 16, pp. 1899–1905).

23   Allegri, M, Montella, S, Salici, F, Valente, A, Marchesini, M, Compagnone, C, Baciarello, M, Manferdini, ME & Fanelli, G. (2016). 'Mechanisms of low back pain: A guide for diagnosis and therapy'. *F1000Research* (vol. 5, p. 1530).

24   Waddell. (2004). *The Back Pain Revolution*, p. 52.

25   Waddell. (2004). *The Back Pain Revolution*, p. 53.

26   Dandy, WE. (1942). 'Concealed ruptured intervertebral disks: A plea for the elimination of contrast mediums in diagnosis'. *Journal of the American Medical Association* (vol. 117, no. 10, pp. 821–23).

27   Brown, T, Nemiah, JC, Barr, JS & Barry, H, Jr. (1954). 'Psychologic factors in low-back pain'. *New England Journal of Medicine* (vol. 251, no. 4, pp. 123–28).

28   Hadler, NM. (2009). *Stabbed in the Back: Confronting Back Pain in an Overtreated Society*. Chapel Hill: University of North Carolina Press, p. 10.

29   O'Sullivan, P. (2012). 'It's time for change with the management of non-specific chronic low back pain'. *British Journal of Sports Medicine* (vol. 46, no. 4, pp. 224–27).

30   Brinjikji, W, Diehn, FE, Jarvik, JG, Carr, CM, Kallmes, DF, Murad, MH & Luetmer, PH. (2015). 'MRI findings of disc degeneration are more prevalent in adults with low back pain than in asymptomatic controls: A systematic review and meta-analysis'. *American Journal of Neuroradiology* (vol. 36, no. 12, pp. 2394–99).

31   Knezevic, NN, Candido, KD, Vlaeyen, JWS, Van Zundert, J & Cohen, SP. (2021). 'Low back pain'. *Lancet* (vol. 398, no. 10294, pp. 78–92).

32   Juch, JNS, Maas, ET, Ostelo, RW, Groeneweg, JG, Kallewaard, J-W, Koes, BW, Verhagen, AP, van Dongen, JM, Huygen, FJPM & van Tulder, MW. (2017). 'Effect of radiofrequency denervation on pain intensity among patients with chronic low back pain'. *JAMA* (vol. 318, no. 1, p. 68).

33   Knezevic et al. (2021). 'Low back pain'.

34   Carragee, EJ, Lincoln, T, Parmar, VS & Alamin, T. (2006). 'A gold standard evaluation of the "discogenic pain" diagnosis as determined by provocative discography'. *Spine* (vol. 31, no. 18, pp. 2115–23).

35   Carragee, EJ, Alamin, TF, Miller, JL & Carragee, JM. (2005). 'Discographic, MRI and psychosocial determinants of low back pain disability and remission: A prospective study in subjects with benign persistent back pain'. *Spine Journal* (vol. 5, no. 1, pp. 24–35).

36   Carragee, EJ, Don, AS, Hurwitz, EL, Cuellar, JM, Carrino, J & Herzog, R. (2009). '2009 ISSLS prize winner: Does discography cause accelerated progression of degeneration changes in the lumbar disc?' *Spine* (vol. 34, no. 21, pp. 2338–45).

37   'The evidence on discography from the Stanford discography project'. (2009). *The Back Letter* (vol. 24, no. 7, p. 82).

38   Hartvigsen, J, Hancock, MJ, Kongsted, A, Louw, Q, Ferreira, ML, Genevay, S, Hoy, D, Karppinen, J, Pransky, G, Sieper, J, Smeets, RJ, Underwood, M, Buchbinder, R, Hartvigsen, J, Cherkin, D, Foster, NE, Maher, CG, &Underwood, M, on behalf of the Lancet Low Back Pain Series Working Group. (2018). 'What low back pain is and why we need to pay attention'. *Lancet* (vol. 391, no. 10137, pp. 2356–67).

4   Too much medicine
1   Honeyman, PT & Jacobs EA. (1996)' Effects of culture on back pain in Australian Aboriginals'. *Spine* (vol. 21, no. 7, pp. 841–43).
2   Lin, IB, O'Sullivan, PB, Coffin, JA, Mak, DB, Toussaint, S & Straker, LM. (2013). 'Disabling chronic low back pain as an iatrogenic disorder: A qualitative study in Aboriginal Australians'. *BMJ Open* (vol. 3, no. 4, p. e002654).
3   Barker, S. (2016). 'The difficult problem: Chronic pain and the politics of care'. *Australian Quarterly*.
4   Lin et al. (2013). 'Disabling chronic low back pain as an iatrogenic disorder'.
5   Bui, Q, Doescher, M, Takeuchi, D & Taylor, V. (2010). 'Immigration, acculturation and chronic back and neck problems among Latino-Americans'. *Journal of Immigrant and Minority Health* (vol. 13, no. 2, pp. 194–201).
6   Henschke, N, Lorenz, E, Pokora, R, Michaleff, ZA, Quartey, JNA & Oliveira, VC. (2016). 'Understanding cultural influences on back pain and back pain research'. *Best. Prac. Res. Clin. Rheumatol.* (vol. 30, no. 6, pp. 1037–1049).
7   Lynch, ME, Craig, KD & Peng, PWH. (eds). (2010). *Clinical Pain Management: A Practical Guide.* 1st edn, Wiley.
8   Williams, CM, Maher, CG, Hancock, MJ, McAuley, JH, McLachlan, AJ, Britt, H, Fahridin, S, Harrison, C & Latimer, J. (2010). 'Low back pain and best practice care: A survey of general practice physicians'. *Archives of Internal Medicine* (vol. 170, no. 3, pp. 271–77).
9   Henschke, N, Maher, CG, Refshauge, KM, Herbert, RD, Cumming, RG, Bleasel, J, York, J, Das, A & McAuley, JH. (2009). 'Prevalence of and screening for serious spinal pathology in patients presenting to primary care settings with acute low back pain'. *Arthritis Rheum.* (vol. 60, no. 10, pp. 3072–80).
10   Kendrick, D, Fielding, K, Bentley, E, Kerslake, R, Miller, P & Pringle, M. (2001). 'Radiography of the lumbar spine in primary care patients with low back pain: Randomised controlled trial'. *BMJ* (vol. 322, no. 7283, pp. 400–405).
11   Webster, BS, Bauer, AZ, Choi, Y, Cifuentes, M. & Pransky, GS. (2013). 'Iatrogenic consequences of early magnetic resonance imaging in acute, work-related, disabling low back pain'. *Spine* (vol. 38, no. 22, pp. 1939–46).
12   Webster, B.S, Choi, Y, Bauer, AZ, Cifuentes, M & Pransky, G. (2014). 'The cascade of medical services and associated longitudinal costs due to nonadherent magnetic resonance imaging for low back pain'. *Spine* (vol. 39, no. 17, pp. 1433–40).
13   Jarvik, JG, Hollingworth, W, Martin, B, Emerson, S S, Gray, DT, Overman, S, Robinson, D, Staiger, T, Wessbecher, F, Sullivan, SD,

Kreuter, W & Deyo, RA. (2003). 'Rapid magnetic resonance imaging vs radiographs for patients with low back pain'. *JAMA* (vol. 289, no. 21, p. 2810).

14   Harris, IA & Dao, ATT. (2009). 'Trends of spinal fusion surgery in Australia: 1997 to 2006'. *ANZ Journal of Surgery* (vol. 79, no. 11, pp. 783–88).

15   Jacobs, JC, Jarvik, JG, Chou, R, Boothroyd, D, Lo, J, Nevedal, A & Barnett, PG. (2020). 'Observational study of the downstream consequences of inappropriate MRI of the lumbar spine'. *Journal of General Internal Medicine* (vol. 35, no. 12, pp. 3605–12).

16   Herzog, R, Elgort, DR, Flanders, AE & Moley, PJ. (2017). 'Variability in diagnostic error rates of 10 MRI centers performing lumbar spine MRI examinations on the same patient within a 3-week period'. *Spine Journal* (vol. 17, no. 4, pp. 554–61).

17   Harris, IA. (2016). *Surgery, the Ultimate Placebo: A Surgeon Cuts through the Evidence*. Sydney: NewSouth, p. 217.

5   'Good posture' – and other back myths

1   Gilman, SL. (2014). '"Stand up straight": Notes toward a history of posture'. *Journal of Medical Humanities* (vol. 35, no. 1, pp. 57–83).

2   Richards, KV, Beales, DJ, Smith, AJ, O'Sullivan, PB & Straker, LM. (2016). 'Neck posture clusters and their association with biopsychosocial factors and neck pain in Australian adolescents'. *Physical Therapy* (vol. 96, no. 10, pp. 1576–87).

3   Mahmoud, NF, Hassan, K.A, Abdelmajeed, SF, Moustafa, IM & Silva, AG. (2019). 'The relationship between forward head posture and neck pain: A systematic review and meta-analysis'. *Current Reviews in Musculoskeletal Medicine* (vol. 12, no. 4, pp. 562–77).

4   Swain, CTV, Pan, F, Owen, PJ, Schmidt, H & Belavy, DL. (2020). 'No consensus on causality of spine postures or physical exposure and low back pain: A systematic review of systematic reviews'. *Journal of Biomechanics* (vol. 102, p. 109312).

5   Roffey, D. M., Wai, E. K., Bishop, P., Kwon, B. K., & Dagenais, S. (2010). Causal assessment of awkward occupational postures and low back pain: Results of a systematic review. *Spine Journal* (vol. 10, no. 1, pp. 89–99).

6   Shape, M. 'The #1 reason you should care about your abs – that sas nothing to do with a six-pack'. Shape, 5 May 2023, <www.shape.com/fitness/tips/why-its-so-important-have-core-strength>.

7   Erkal, MM. (2017). 'The cultural history of the corset and gendered body in social and literary landscapes'. *European Journal of Language and Literature* (vol. 3, no. 3, pp. 109–18).

8   Hodges, PW & Richardson, CA. 'Altered trunk muscle recruitment in people with low back pain with upper limb movement at different

speeds'. *Archives of Physical Medicine and Rehabilitation* (vol. 80, no. 9, Sept. 1999, pp. 1005–12).

9   Gubler, D, Mannion, AF, Schenk, P, Gorelick, M, Helbling, D, Gerber, H, Toma, V & Sprott, H. (2010). 'Ultrasound tissue doppler imaging reveals no delay in abdominal muscle feed-forward activity during rapid arm movements in patients with chronic low back pain'. *Spine* (vol. 35, no. 16, pp. 1506–13).

10 Wang, X-Q, Zheng, J-J, Yu, Z-W, Bi, X, Lou, S-J, Liu, J, Cai, B, Hua, Y-H, Wu, M, Wei, M-L, Shen, H-M, Chen, Y, Pan, Y-J, Xu, G-H & Chen, P-J. (2012). 'A meta-analysis of core stability exercise versus general exercise for chronic low back pain'. *PLoS ONE* (vol. 7, no. 12, p. e52082); Smith, BE, Littlewood, C & May, S. (2014). 'An update of stabilisation exercises for low back pain: A systematic review with meta-analysis'. *BMC Musculoskeletal Disorders* (vol. 15, no. 1).

11 Ramin, C.J. (2017). *Crooked: Outwitting the Back Pain Industry and Getting on the Road to Recovery.* 1st edn. New York: Harper, p. 48.

12 'A Tribute to Alf Nachemson – The Spine: Interview'. (2007). *The Back Letter* (vol. 22, no. 2, p. 13).

13 'A Tribute to Alf Nachemson'. (2007).

14 Nachemson, A. (1960). 'Lumbar intradiscal pressure: Experimental studies on post-mortem material'. *Acta Orthopaedica Scandinavica. Suppl.* (vol. 43, 1960, pp. 1–104).

15 Nachemson, A. (1965). 'The effect of forward leaning on lumbar intradiscal pressure'. *Acta Orthopaedica Scandinavica* (vol. 35, no. 1–4, pp. 314–28).

16 Saraceni, N, Kent, P, Ng, L, Campbell, A, Straker, L & O'Sullivan, P. (2020). 'To flex or not to flex? Is there a relationship between lumbar spine flexion during lifting and low back pain? A systematic review with meta-analysis'. *Journal of Orthopaedic Sports Physical Therapy* (vol. 50, no. 3, pp. 121–30).

17 'A Tribute to Alf Nachemson – The Spine: Interview'. (2007). *The Back Letter* (vol. 22, no. 2, p. 13).

18 Darlow, B, Perry, M, Stanley, J, Mathieson, F, Melloh, M, Baxter, GD & Dowell, A. (2014). 'Cross-sectional survey of attitudes and beliefs about back pain in New Zealand'. *BMJ Open* (vol. 4, no. 5, p. e004725).

19 Jensen, MP. 'Hypnosis for chronic pain management: A new hope'. *Pain* (vol. 146, no. 3, Dec. 2009, p. 235).

20 Rizzo, RRN, Medeiros, FC, Pires, LG, Pimenta, RM, McAuley, JH, Jensen, MP & Costa, LOP. (2018). 'Hypnosis enhances the effects of pain education in patients with chronic nonspecific low back pain: A randomized controlled trial'. *Journal of Pain* (vol. 19, no. 10, p. 1103. e1 – 1103.e9).

21 Ng, SK, Cicuttini, FM, Wang, Y, Wluka, AE, Fitzgibbon, B & Urquhart, DM. (2016). 'Negative beliefs about low back pain are associated with

persistent high intensity low back pain'. *Psychology, Health & Medicine* (vol. 22, no. 7, pp. 790–99).

22   Buchbinder, R & Harris, IA. (2021). *Hippocrasy: How Doctors Are Betraying Their Oath.* Sydney: NewSouth, p. 167.

23   Buchbinder, & Harris. *Hippocrasy*, p. 168.

6   Pain and profit

1   Deyo, RA, Mirza, SK, Turner, JA & Martin, BI. (2009). 'Overtreating chronic back pain: Time to back off?' *Journal of the American Board of Family Medicine* (vol. 22, no. 1, pp. 62–68).

2   Hanscom, D. (2019). *Do You Really Need Spine Surgery?: Take Control with a Surgeon's Advice.* Oakland: Vertus Press, p. 124.

3   Harris, IA & Dao, ATT. (2009). 'Trends of spinal fusion surgery in Australia: 1977 to 2006.' ANZ Journal of Surgery, <https://doi.org/10.1111/j.1445-2197.2009.05095.x>.

4   Hadler, NM. (2009). *Stabbed in the Back: Confronting Back Pain in an Overtreated Society.* Chapel Hill: University of North Carolina Press, p. 10.

5   Deyo, RA. (2014). *Watch Your Back! How the Back Pain Industry Is Costing Us More and Giving Us Less, and What You Can Do to Inform and Empower Yourself in Seeking Treatment.* Ithaca: ILR Press, p. 97.

6   Harris, IA & Buchbinder, R. (2013). 'Time to reconsider steroid injections in the spine?' *Medical Journal of Australia* (vol. 199, no. 4, pp. 237–37).

7   Ramin, CJ. (2017). *Crooked: Outwitting the Back Pain Industry and Getting on the Road to Recovery.* 1st edn. New York: Harper, p. 56.

8   Harris & Buchbinder. (2013). 'Time to reconsider steroid injections in the spine?'

9   Staal, JB, de Bie, R, de Vet, HCW, Hildebrandt, J & Nelemans, P. (2008). 'Injection therapy for subacute and chronic low-back pain'. *Cochrane Database of Systematic Reviews.*

10   Chou, R, Hashimoto, R, Friedly, J, Fu, R, Bougatsos, C, Dana, T, Sullivan, SD & Jarvik, J. (2015). 'Epidural corticosteroid injections for radiculopathy and spinal stenosis: A systematic review and meta-analysis'. *Annals of Internal Medicine* (vol. 163, no. 5, pp. 373–81).

11   Oliveira, CB, Maher, CG, Ferreira, ML, Hancock, MJ, Oliveira, VC, McLachlan, AJ, Koes, BW, Ferreira, PH, Cohen, SP & Pinto, RZ. (2020). 'Epidural corticosteroid injections for lumbosacral radicular pain'. *Cochrane Database of Systematic Reviews* (no. 4).

12   Deyo. (2014). *Watch Your Back!*, p. 100.

13   Heary, RF. (2001). 'Intradiscal electrothermal annuloplasty: The IDET procedure'. *Journal of Spinal Disorders* (vol. 14, no. 4, pp. 353–60).

14   Wegener, B, Rieskamp, K, Büttner, A, Habiyambere, V, von Schultze-Pellangahr, C, Schaffer, V, Jansson, V & Birkenmaier, C. (2012).

'Experimental evaluation of the risk of extradiscal thermal damage in intradiscal electrothermal therapy (IDET)'. *Pain Physician* (vol. 15, no. 1, pp. E99–106).

15   Saal, JS & Saal, JA. (2000). 'Management of chronic discogenic low back pain with a thermal intradiscal catheter: A preliminary report'. *Spine* (vol. 25, no. 3, pp. 382–88).

16   Hadler. (2009). *Stabbed in the Back*, p. 80.

17   Hadler. (2009). *Stabbed in the Back*, p. 80.

18   'Back Break'. Forbes, 12 August 2002, www.forbes.com/ forbes/2002/0812/123.html>.

19   Freeman, BJC. (2006). 'IDET: A critical appraisal of the evidence'. *European Spine Journal* (vol. 15, pp. 448–57).

20   Russo, M, Santarelli, D, Wright, R & Gilligan, C. (2021). 'A history of the development of radiofrequency neurotomy'. *Journal of Pain Research* (vol. 14, pp. 3897–3907).

21   Leclaire, R, Fortin, L, Lambert, R, Bergeron, YM & Rossignol, M. (2001). 'Radiofrequency facet joint denervation in the treatment of low back pain: A placebo-controlled clinical trial to assess efficacy'. *Spine* (vol. 26, no. 13, pp. 1411–16).

22   Maas, ET, Ostelo, RWJG, Niemisto, L, Jousimaa, J, Hurri, H, Malmivaara, A & van Tulder, MW. (2015). 'Radiofrequency denervation for chronic low back pain'. *Cochrane Library*.

23   Hadler. (2009). *Stabbed in the Back*, p. 81.

7   Big pharma

1   Smith, PA. 'How an island in the Antipodes became the world's leading supplier of licit opioids'. *Pacific Standard*, 24 July 2019, <psmag.com/ ideas/opioids-limiting-the-legal-supply-wont-stop-the-overdose-crisis>.

2   Thomas, K & Hsu, T. 'Johnson & Johnson's brand falters over its role in the opioid crisis.' *New York Times*, 27 August 2019.

3   Whoriskey, P. 'How Johnson & Johnson companies used a "super poppy" to make narcotics for America's most abused opioid pills'. *Washington Post*, 26 March 2020, <www.washingtonpost.com/ graphics/2020/business/opioid-crisis-johnson-and-johnson-tasmania-poppy/>.

4   'How Australia's smallest state wound up in the middle of America's biggest drug crisis'. *ABC News*, 12 October 2019.

5   Pathan, H & Williams, J. (2012). 'Basic opioid pharmacology: An update'. *British Journal of Pain* (vol. 6, no. 1, pp. 11–16).

6   Gelineau, K, 'Opioid Crisis Is Not Just an American Problem'. Australian Financial Review, 6 September 2019, <www.afr.com/ companies/healthcare-and-fitness/opioid-crisis-is-not-just-an-american-problem-20190905-p52oef>.

7   Alpert, A, Evans, W, Lieber, EMJ & Powell, D. (2019). *Origins of the Opioid Crisis and Its Enduring Impacts*. Cambridge, MA: National Bureau of Economic Research.

8   Brownstein, M.J. (1993). 'A brief history of opiates, opioid peptides, and opioid receptors'. *Proceedings of the National Academy of Sciences* (vol. 90, no. 12, pp. 5391–93).

9   'From cough medicine to deadly addiction: A century of heroin and drug-abuse policy.' (1999). Yale Medicine Magazine, <medicine.yale. edu/news/yale-medicine-magazine/article/from-cough-medicine-to-deadly-addiction-a-century/>.

10   Gelineau, K. 'Surging prescriptions, deaths: Australia faces opioid crisis.' *AP News in partnership with Pulitzer Center on Crisis Reporting*, 6 September 2019, <pulitzercenter.org/stories/surging-prescriptions-deaths-australia-faces-opioid-crisis>.

11   Keefe, PR. 'The family that built an empire of pain'. *New Yorker*, 23 October 2017, <www.newyorker.com/magazine/2017/10/30/the-family-that-built-an-empire-of-pain>.

12   Marks, JH. (2020). 'Lessons from corporate influence in the opioid epidemic: Toward a norm of separation'. *Journal of Bioethical Inquiry* (vol. 17, no. 2, pp. 173–89).

13   Porter, J & Jick, H. (1980). 'Addiction rare in patients treated with narcotics'. *New England Journal of Medicine* (vol. 302, no. 2, p. 123).

14   Deyo, RA, Von Korff, M & Duhrkoop, D. (2015). 'Opioids for low back pain'. *BMJ* (vol. 350, p. g6380).

15   Tomazin, F. 'Australia's opioid crisis: Deaths rise as companies encourage doctors to prescribe'. *The Age*, 4 February 2020, <www. theage.com.au/national/australia-s-opioid-crisis-deaths-rise-as-companies-encourage-doctors-to-prescribe-20200203-p53x72.html>.

16   Van Zee, A. (2009). 'The promotion and marketing of OxyContin: Commercial triumph, public health tragedy'. *American Journal of Public Health* (vol. 99, no. 2, pp. 221–27).

17   Macy, B. (2018). *Dopesick: Dealers, Doctors, and the Drug Company That Addicted America*. 1st edn. New York: Little, Brown & Co, p. 94.

18   Krebs, EE, Gravely, A, Nugent, S, Jensen, AC, DeRonne, B, Goldsmith, E.S, Kroenke, K, Bair, MJ & Noorbaloochi, S. (2018).' Effect of opioid vs nonopioid medications on pain-related function in patients with chronic back pain or hip or knee osteoarthritis pain: The SPACE Randomized Clinical Trial'. *JAMA* (vol. 319, no. 9, pp. 872–82).

8   Spinal surgery

1   Harris, IA. (2016). *Surgery, the Ultimate Placebo: A Surgeon Cuts through the Evidence*. Sydney: NewSouth, p. 131.

2   Virk, S, Qureshi, S & Sandhu, H. (2020). 'History of spinal fusion: Where we came from and where we are going'. *HSS Journal* (vol. 16, no. 2, pp. 137–42).

3   Atkinson, L & Zacest, A. (2016). 'Surgical management of low back pain'. *Medical Journal of Australia* (vol. 204, no. 8).

4   Zaina, F, Tomkins-Lane, C, Carragee, E & Negrini, S. (2016). 'Surgical versus non-surgical treatment for lumbar spinal stenosis'. *Cochrane Database of Systematic Reviews* (no. 1).

5   Harris, IA, Traeger, A, Stanford, R, Maher, CG & Buchbinder, R. (2018). 'Lumbar spine fusion: What is the evidence?: Lumbar fusion'. *Internal Medicine Journal* (vol. 48, no. 12, pp. 1430–34).

6   McMillan, JS, Jones, K, Forgan, L, Busija, L, Carey, RPL, de Silva, AM & Phillips, MG. (2022). 'Lumbar spinal fusion surgery outcomes in a cohort of injured workers in the Victorian workers' compensation system'. *ANZ Journal of Surgery* (vol. 92, no. 3, pp. 481–86).

7   Lewin, AM, Fearnside, M, Kuru, R, Jonker, BP, Naylor, JM., Sheridan, M & Harris, IA. (2021). 'Rates, costs, return to work and reoperation following spinal surgery in a workers' compensation cohort in New South Wales, 2010–2018: A cohort study using administrative data'. *BMC Health Services Research* (vol. 21, no. 1, p. 955).

8   Murrey, D, Janssen, M, Delamarter, R, Goldstein, J, Zigler, J, Tay, B & Darden, B. (2009). 'Results of the prospective, randomized, controlled multicenter Food and Drug Administration investigational device exemption study of the ProDisc-C total disc replacement versus anterior discectomy and fusion for the treatment of 1-Level symptomatic cervical disc disease'. *Spine Journal* (vol. 9, no. 4, pp. 275–86).

9   Daniell, JR & Osti, OL. (2018). 'Failed back surgery syndrome: A review article'. *Asian Spine Journal* (vol. 12, no. 2, pp. 372–79).

10   Thomson, S. 'Failed back surgery syndrome – definition, epidemiology and demographics'. *British Journal of Pain* (vol. 7, no. 1, pp. 56–59).

11   Harris, IA. (2016). *Surgery, the Ultimate Placebo*, p. 1.

9   The new science of pain

1   Moayedi, M & Davis, KD. (2013). 'Theories of pain: From specificity to gate control'. *Journal of Neurophysiology* (vol. 109, no. 1, pp. 5–12).

2   Biegler, P. (2023). Why Does It Still Hurt?: How the Power of Knowledge Can Overcome Chronic Pain. Melbourne: Scribe Publications, p. 28.

3   Melzack, R & Wall, PD. 'Pain Mechanisms: A New Theory: A Gate Control System Modulates Sensory Input from the Skin before It Evokes Pain Perception and Response', Science, November 1965 (vol. 150, no. 3699, pp. 971–79, <https://doi.org/10.1126/science.150.3699.971>.

4   Butler, DS & Moseley, GL. (2019). *Explain Pain*. 2nd edn. Adelaide: Noigroup Publications, p. 37.

5   Butler, DS & Lorimer Moseley, G. (2019). Explain Pain, p. 17.

6   Bayer, TL, Baer, PE & Early, C. (1991). 'Situational and psychophysiological factors in psychologically induced pain'. *Pain* (vol. 44, no. 1, pp. 45–50).

7   *New Insights from Pain Neuroscience – Dr Tasha Stanton*, <www.youtube.com/watch?v=ZWvyLJkBrLY>.

8   Stanton, TR, Moseley, GL, Wong, AYL & Kawchuk, GN. (2017). 'Feeling stiffness in the back: A protective perceptual inference in chronic back pain'. *Scientific Reports* (vol. 7, no. 1, p. 9681).

9   *New Insights from Pain Neuroscience.*

10   *Pain, the Brain and Your Amazing Protectometer – Lorimer Moseley*, <www.youtube.com/watch?v=lCF1_Fs00nM>.

11   *Pain, the Brain and Your Amazing Protectometer.*

12   Meldrum, ML. (2003). 'A capsule history of pain management'. *JAMA* (vol. 290, no. 18, pp. 2470–75).

13   Buchbinder, R & Harris, IA. (2021). *Hippocrasy: How Doctors Are Betraying Their Oath*. Sydney: NewSouth, p. 20.

14   Barker, S. (2016). 'The difficult problem: Chronic pain and the politics of care'. *Australian Quarterly.*

10   The mind–body–back connection

1   Chou, R & Shekelle, P. (2010). 'Will this patient develop persistent disabling low back pain?' *JAMA* (vol. 303, no. 13, pp. 1295–1302).

2   Chou & Shekelle. (2010). 'Will this patient develop persistent disabling low back pain?'

3   Segerstrom, SC & Miller, GE. (2004). 'Psychological stress and the human immune system: A meta-analytic study of 30 years of inquiry'. *Psychological Bulletin* (vol. 130, no. 4, pp. 601–30).

4   Carnegie Mellon University. (2012). *Science Daily*. 'How stress influences disease: Study reveals inflammation as the culprit'.

5   Dario, AB, Kamper, SJ, O'Keeffe, M, Zadro, J, Lee, H, Wolfenden, L & Williams, CM. (2019). 'Family history of pain and risk of musculoskeletal pain in children and adolescents: A systematic review and meta-analysis'. *Pain* (vol. 160, no. 11, pp. 2430–39).

6   Sturgeon, JA & Zautra, A.J. (2010). 'Resilience: a new paradigm for adaptation to chronic pain'. *Current Pain and Headache Reports* (vol. 14, no. 2, p. 105–12).

11   Overcoming fear

1   Pontzer, H. (2018). 'Energy constraint as a novel mechanism linking exercise and health'. *Physiology* (vol. 33, no. 6, pp. 384–93).

2   Costa, N, Smits, EJ, Kasza, J, Salomoni, S, Rodriguez-Romero, B, Ferreira, ML, Hodges, PW. (2022). 'Are objective measures of sleep and sedentary behaviours related to low back pain flares?' *Pain* (vol. 163, no. 9, pp. 1829–37).

3   Foster, NE, Anema, JR, Cherkin, D, Chou, R, Cohen, SP, Gross, DP, Ferreira, PH, Fritz, JM, Koes, BW, Peul, W, Turner, JA, Maher, CG., on behalf of the Lancet Low Back Pain Series Working Group. (2018). 'Prevention and treatment of low back pain: Evidence, challenges, and promising directions'. Lancet (vol. 391, no. 10137, pp. 2368–83).

4   Gloster, AT, Walder, N, Levin, ME, Twohig, MP & Karekla, M. (2020). 'The empirical status of acceptance and commitment therapy: A review of meta-analyses'. *Journal of Contextual Behavioral Science* (vol. 18, pp. 181–92).

5   Côté, P. (2020). 'A united statement of the global chiropractic research community against the pseudoscientific claim that chiropractic care boosts immunity'. *Chiropractic & Manual Therapies* (vol. 28, no. 1, p. 21).

12   A different approach to back pain

1   Pontzer, H. (2018). 'Energy constraint as a novel mechanism linking exercise and health'. *Physiology* (vol. 33, no. 6, pp. 384–93).

2   Costa, N, Smitz, EJ, Kasza, J, Solomon, S, Rodriguez-Romano, B, Ferreira, ML, Hodges, PW. (2002). 'Are objective measures of sleep and sedentary behaviours related to low back pain states?' Pain (vol. 163, no.0, pp. 1829–37).

3   Foster, NE, Anema, JR, Cherkin, D, Chou, R, Cohen, SP, Gross, DP, Ferreira, PH, Fritz, JM, Koes, BW. Peul, W, Turner, JA, Maher, CG., on behalf of the Lancet Low Back Pain Series Working Group. (2018). 'Prevention and treatment of low back pain: Evidence, challenges, and promising directions'. Lancet (vol. 391, no. 10137, pp. 2368–83).

4   Milzoff, R. 'For the World's Best Male Ballet Dancer, Injury Led to Artistic Rebirth'.Vulture, 18 May 2017, <www.vulture.com/2017/05/for-david-hallberg-injury-led-to-artistic-rebirth.html>.

5   Thompson, C. 'The Rebirth of David Hallberg'. Dance Magazine, 21 May 2017, < www.dancemagazine.com/the-rebirth-of-david-hallberg/>.

6   Gloster, A. T., Walder, N., Levin, M. E., Twohig, M. P., & Karekla, M. (2020). The empirical status of acceptance and commitment therapy: A review of meta-analyses. *Journal of Contextual Behavioral Science* (vol. 18, pp. 181–92).

7   Ho, EK-Y, Chen, L, Simic, M, Ashton-James, CE, Comachio, J, Wang, DXM, Hayden, JA, Ferreira, ML & Ferreira, PH. (2022). 'Psychological interventions for chronic, non-specific low back pain: Systematic

review with network meta-analysis'. BMJ, 30 March 2022, <376, e067718. https://doi.org/10.1136/bmj-2021-067718>.

8   Côté, P. (2020). A united statement of the global chiropractic research community against the pseudoscientific claim that chiropractic care boosts immunity. *Chiropractic & Manual Therapies* (vol. 28, no. 1, p. 21).

9   Watson, JA, Ryan, CG, Cooper, L, Ellington, D, Whittle, R, Lavender, M, Dixon, J, Atkinson, G, Cooper, K, Martin, D. (2019) 'Pain neuroscience education for Adults with chronic musculoskeletal pain: A mixed-methods systematic review and meta-analysis.' The Journal of Pain (vol. 20, no. 10, p. 1140.e1-1140.e22).

10   Wood, L, & Hendrick, P. (2019) 'A systematic review and meta-analysis of pain neuroscience education for chronic low back pain: Short- and long-term outcomes of pain and disability.' European Journal of Pain (vol. 23, no. 2, pp. 234–49. PubMed), <https://doi.org/10.1002/ejp.1314>.

11   Kent, P, Haines, T, O'Sullivan, P, Smith, A, Campbell, A, Schutze, R, Attwell, S, Caneiro, JP, Laird, R, O'Sullivan, K, McGregor, A, Hartvigsen, J, Lee, D-CA, Vickery, A, Hancock, M & RESTORE trial team. (2023). 'Cognitive functional therapy with or without movement sensor biofeedback versus usual care for chronic, disabling low back pain (Restore): A randomised, controlled, three-arm, parallel group, phase 3, clinical trial'. *Lancet*, S0140-6736(23)00441-5 <https://doi.org/10.1016/S0140-6736(23)00441-5>.

Index